The Real Life
of a
Surgeon

Candid Stories Along the Path
from Student to Veteran Doctor

The
Real Life

of a
Surgeon

Arthur W. Perry, MD, FACS

Editor

KAPLAN
PUBLISHING

New York

© 2009 Kaplan, Inc.

Published by Kaplan Publishing, a division of Kaplan, Inc.
1 Liberty Plaza, 24th Floor
New York, NY 10006

Library of Congress Cataloging-in-Publication Data

The real life of a surgeon / Arthur Perry, editor.
    p. ; cm.
ISBN 978-1-60714-117-4
1. Surgery--Popular works. I. Perry, Arthur W.
[DNLM: 1. General Surgery--Personal Narratives. WZ 112.5.S8 R288 2009]
RD31.3.R43 2009
617--dc22

                                    2009023217

Printed in the United States

10 9 8 7 6 5 4 3 2 1   4491 1906 1/11

ISBN-13: 978-1-60714-117-4

This book is dedicated to my wife, Bedonna, and my children, Benjamin, Meredith, and Julia, and to my parents, Harriet and Dr. Michael Perry. They have experienced, firsthand, the Real Life of a Surgeon.

Contents

Introduction

Arthur W. Perry, MD, FACS

Surgery is the most aggressive discipline in medicine. In medical school, you always knew who would go into surgery. Usually not the most cerebral (they went into neurology or oncology) and not the edgy kids (they went into psychiatry). The nurturing ones? They went into pediatrics. And the computer geeks went into radiology so they could be surrounded with technology. The kids with ADD went into surgery. They needed immediate results. Diseases can be cured in an afternoon with surgery. And even within surgery, the psychologists know that the carpenters go into orthopedics and the creative ones go into plastic surgery.

Surgery is simultaneously glamorous and down-and-dirty. Dr. Hawkeye Pierce in *M*A*S*H* typified the surgeon: self-assured, aggressive, and somewhat cocky. You may not like these qualities in your spouse or tennis partner, but they're exactly what you want in your surgeon. But how did your surgeon get that way? Genetics or environment? Probably a combination of the two.

The surgical training program is known as the most arduous in all of medicine. After four years of college and four years of medical school, surgeons train for five to eight years in grueling residency programs. Following residency, board certification requires passing both written and oral exams. And when that's done, if you're motivated, you apply and interview to become a Fellow of the American College of Surgeons. Those who achieve this status wear the "FACS" proudly after their names. You don't go into surgery if you're lazy, if you're not willing to work longer and harder than any other doctor in the hospital.

Depending on the number of years following medical school graduation, trainees are called interns, residents, or fellows. These surgeons-in-training face schedules as grueling as the notorious "every other night," routinely clocking in over a hundred hours a week in the hospital. At a cocktail party, ask a surgeon if he ever fell asleep in the operating room after being up the entire night before. I don't know many who haven't. Thank goodness for the new laws that limit residents' hours, protecting patients.

The mentality of surgeons is often shaped by this demanding schedule, as well as by the treatment they receive from their superiors—fully trained surgeons called *attendings.* Expressions like "surgeons eat their young" and "beaten resident syndrome" describe some of the "fun" times during residency. And along with the merciless schedule, residents have to deal with the infamous *pyramid.* That's a general surgery residency program that accepts sixteen newly minted doctors, for instance, but graduates only four. The other twelve are "cut" from the program and either go into surgical subspecialties or find another field, such as anesthesiology. Makes for a collegial atmosphere, don't you think?

It takes a certain strong personality to take knife in hand and slice through human tissue, knowing that the patient's life and limbs are, quite literally, in your hands. A good surgeon knows *when* to operate and *how* to operate. He or she must possess medical knowledge and good judgment. Like the "chops" of a musician, a surgeon must have "hands." Klutzes can't go into surgery.

This book brings you into the world of real surgeons. Not those television characters with tailored attire who scrub their hands with their masks down so you can see their mouths move. Real surgeons who handle scalpels, clamps, sutures, lasers, and now sometimes robots every day. Real surgeons with marking ink on their hands and crinkled, faded scrubs. Many of the writers of this book are surgeons with whom I have worked at different phases of my career, and most were handpicked to share their stories. These are the leaders in the surgical world, and I hope that by reading their stories you'll understand why they're regarded as the world's experts.

You'll read about how the Chief of Plastic Surgery at Columbia and Cornell, **Dr. Robert Grant,** saved a patient's life by cracking open his chest right there in the patient's hospital room to perform cardiac massage. Imagine the look on the face of the patient in the next bed! You'll read about how the world's foremost liver surgeon, **Dr. Yuman Fong**, vice-chairman of surgery at Memorial Sloan-Kettering, saved the life of a little girl with a cancer growing into her heart. (Have your handkerchiefs ready.) And when you've recovered from that story, read about how **Dr. Jim Goydos**, director of the melanoma center at Robert Wood Johnson Medical School, went one up on television doctor House and figured out how to cure a patient with a cancer so rare that most doctors don't know it exists.

You'll marvel at how Rush University ophthalmologist **Dr. Ronald Weiss's** surgical skills, against all odds, restored vision to a Somalian refugee. And when you think you have heard it all, read how Robert Wood Johnson cardiac surgeon **Dr. Mark Anderson** saved the life of a fellow surgeon by transplanting his heart during a life-and-death emergency. **Your editor** will then bring you into the smells and sounds of the world's largest burn center, giving you more reason to check the batteries in your smoke detectors. I will then tell you why I buck the "cowboy" image of the surgeon as you read about the patient who taught me to think *before* I cut. In another story, I will let you in on the secrets of my decade as a surgeon on the regulatory board for doctors.

The Real Life of a Surgeon brings you into the lives of some of the most famous surgeons in the world. Texas Heart Institute founder **Dr. Denton Cooley** reveals how he did the first open heart surgery. And for good measure, he tells how he came to perform the first u.s. heart transplant. Then, Breast surgery pioneer **Dr. Susan Love** explains how she battled the male-dominated field of surgery to become a Harvard practitioner, creating an entirely new field within medicine and becoming (one of) the nation's first breast surgeons.

Plastic surgery legend **Dr. Thomas Krizek,** trainer of more chairpersons of plastic surgery than anyone else in the world, gives a lesson about how plastic surgeons have the power to restore a sense of wholeness to patients. Dr. Krizek guided my research during medical school and taught me much of what I know about plastic surgery. An inspiring teacher and surgeon, he teaches and writes in a most entertaining way.

And my chief at Harvard Medical School, **Dr. William Silen,** explains why the best surgeons are more than just technicians. His philosophy, taught to a generation of surgeons, stresses that surgeons are physicians first—healers who also operate.

But surgeons are not just physicians; we're people too. The human side, the personal side, of surgeons is usually hidden from public view. **Dr. Bruce Gewertz,** vascular surgeon and Chairman of Surgery at Cedars-Sinai Medical Center in Los Angeles, shares his own struggles with a rare form of male breast cancer. Moving to the other side of the mirror, doctors-turned-patients discover a personal side of illness, which leads to an uncommon bond with their patients.

Who would have guessed that the surgeon who has the world's largest experience in performing laproscopic band surgery for weight loss would have had the procedure himself? New York University general laparoscopic surgeon **Dr. George Fielding** relates his very personal battle with obesity. But few surgeons have been as close to the "other side" and back as University of Chicago plastic surgeon **Dr. Larry Zachary**, after a careless driver sent him straight into a coma and out of surgery for more than a year. Dr. Zachary's struggle to return to work is inspiring, to say the least. Then, learn from cancer surgeon **Dr. Richard Karl**, former Chairman of Surgery at the University of South Florida, as he lets you in on how his dog taught him something about understanding patients. My four basset hounds enjoyed his story, as you will too.

This is real life, and you'll read how trauma surgeon **Dr. Meghann Kaiser** saved the life of a little boy but wonders if it was really the right thing to do. And you will be simultaneously fascinated and repulsed by neurosurgeon **Dr. Ian Dorward's** story about how he saved the life of a young man with a brain aneurysm not once, but twice. Then enter the OR with **Dr. John Popp**, Harvard neurosurgeon and former Chairman of Surgery at the Albany Medical College, as he saves the life of his childhood hero's wife, bringing her out of a two-year coma! And the sights and sounds of war come alive as you travel to Iraq with military pediatric surgeon **Lt. Col. Christopher Coppola, MD**.

Sometimes surgeons are involved in the creation of life, not just the saving of it—as we learn from in vitro fertilization specialist **Dr. Jane Miller**, as she sorts through mysterious symptoms in a patient determined to get pregnant. We'll hear from New York University vascular surgeon **Neal Cayne, MD,** who saved my own father's life. Dr. Cayne tells how he matured as a person and as a surgeon while up to his elbows in blood in the Bronx, New York. And finally, you'll take a bumpy ride with general surgeon turned burn surgeon turned cosmetic surgeon **Dr. Al Cram** as he navigates the twists and turns of his professional career. I was a part of one of Al's twists at the University of Chicago, as he changed course mid-career.

Almost everyone needs a surgeon eventually. When you visit your surgeon, think of the arduous training, the degree of responsibility that only surgeons, airplane pilots, and military leaders possess, and look carefully at the little wrinkles around their eyes. They have earned every one of them.

As you read through the varied, complex collection of stories in *The Real Life of a Surgeon*, you will begin to understand the thought processes and stresses that are unique to the surgeon's experience. You will journey into the homes, offices, emergency rooms, and operating rooms with some of the best surgeons in the country. And you'll experience their fears and illnesses along with them. Surgery is a dynamic specialty, and the physicians who hold the scalpels are some of the most interesting people you'll ever meet. Find a comfortable chair, fasten your seat belts, and get ready for *The Real Life of a Surgeon*.

LIFE AND DEATH

Neal S. Cayne, MD, FACS

MUCH HAS BEEN WRITTEN about the surgical residency. The long hours without sleep, the seemingly endless flow of patients in and out of the hospital, and the tough way that surgeons have to learn. In a training program, there are certain defining moments all surgeons have that alter the rest of their career: the first life saved and the first life lost. From my days in residency training at the Montefiore Medical Center and Jacobi Hospital in the Bronx, I can clearly remember both.

The Bronx is a gritty part of New York, and that fact provided surgical trainees with a healthy dose of trauma. I was the intern covering the trauma service one evening when a forty-five-year-old man, a husband and father of two teenage girls, got slammed by a Mack truck while driving on the Cross Bronx Expressway. The patient came into the emergency room with a breathing tube already inserted by the ambulance crew, and with unstable vital signs. He was rushed to the operating room with numerous injuries. His aorta, the blood vessel that carries all the blood from the heart to the rest of the body, was torn and massively bleeding in the chest and belly.

When a car stops short, the groceries on the back seat become airborne, hitting the windshield as they continue to travel. The same thing happens inside your body: your organs keep going forward, even after your body has stopped short. And while our bodies are made to withstand the traumas of ten thousand years ago, evolution didn't factor in cars or airplanes. So, when a car goes from sixty miles per hour to zero in a half a second, the fragile blood vessels snap off like twigs on a tree.

My job as the intern that day was to hold a retractor on the aorta while my chief resident worked. As we operated, I remember feeling the warmth of the patient's organs on my gloved hands. As the procedure progressed, the organs cooled to room temperature. I performed my job diligently—not moving a muscle so my chief could save this man's life. But after a while my arm started to become numb and soon my chief resident stopped operating; he looked at the clock on the OR wall, called out the time of death, and told me to come with him.

I was half dazed, half upset, and confused. This was my first death—the first patient who had died with my hands inside his body. I followed my chief resident to a room where the man's wife and two daughters were sitting. The patient had been driving to meet them, and he had never made it to his destination. My chief approached the room, stopped, and turned to me. He told me that this was going to be a good learning experience for me and that I should pay attention. We entered the room and saw the wife and daughters staring at us, wanting to know about their loved one. The now-deceased patient had been a relatively young and otherwise healthy man prior to the accident. My chief looked at the family and paused before saying, "I'm sorry, he didn't make it. He is gone." He then left the room. One daughter looked at me said, "I don't understand. What does he mean?"

At first I was speechless, and I felt myself starting to cry. She asked again. I composed myself as much as I could and tried to explain what had happened. When it registered that their father and husband was dead, all three let out screams and started crying. One daughter started hitting me and screamed, "Why couldn't you save him, why, why?" I said simply, "I'm sorry," and had to leave the room, as I felt myself starting to lose my composure. I left, went to the call room, and began to cry by myself, reflecting on what had just happened. I wasn't there long before another trauma called me to the emergency room, and I started all over again.

As I progressed through my residency, I matured both as a doctor and as a person. As a third-year resident, I remember being called frantically by an intern in the emergency room. I ran to the ER to meet a twenty-one-year-old man who had been shot seven times in the chest and abdomen. He had lost so much blood that soon after arriving in the emergency room, he had no blood pressure at all. As the most senior resident available, I called for the thoracotomy tray. That's the set of instruments that let you open (or *crack*, as we say) a chest to directly control bleeding or even manually pump the heart. As I was taught, I opened his left chest between the fifth and sixth ribs, stuck my hand in, and placed a clamp across the aorta, the main blood vessel in the chest. I then massaged the heart between my hands as others gave the patient uncrossmatched blood and warm fluids. At this point I no longer felt tired, as the adrenaline was flooding through me. We rushed the patient up to the operating room with his chest open and my hand massaging his heart, keeping what little blood he had left in his body flowing to his brain and other organs. Once in the OR, we opened the belly, stopped the abdominal bleeding, and fixed the injured bowel. At this point, my attending arrived. From the story he had received on the telephone, he did not think that the patient would even make it to the operating room. My attending scrubbed in, looked at me, and said, "Congratulations, doc, I think that you just saved this man's life." I looked up at the monitor and saw that the patient's blood pressure was normalizing. When I walked out of the operating room, I felt a euphoria that is almost indescribable. *I had just saved this man's life.* He was someone's son, boyfriend, and brother. This time I was able to tell the family that although in critical condition, their son was alive and could make it. The family hugged me and kissed me and thanked me. He did make it. It took about two months of ICU care, multiple surgeries, and rehab, but he walked out of the hospital.

I am now eight years out of training and a practicing vascular surgeon at the New York University School of Medicine, one of the nation's premier medical institutions. As an academic vascular surgeon, I not only perform surgery but also help teach the next generation of doctors the techniques that will help them save lives. Vascular surgery is undergoing monumental changes, with less-invasive *stents* (new linings inside blood vessels) replacing older, more dangerous procedures. I am happy to be on the cusp of this evolving field.

Overall, my job can be very rewarding but also both emotionally and physically draining. It certainly does have its ups and downs. However, each and every day of work there is always at least one thing that happens that reminds me why I do what I do and why I worked so hard to get here. It could be saving a life or a limb, or it could be as simple as a patient or family member saying thank you for making a difference in their lives. For me, becoming a surgeon was one of the best decisions I have made in my life. Has it been worth all the sacrifice, the years of training? Most certainly. I love my work, and I couldn't see myself doing anything else.

Editor's Note: I met Dr. Cayne three years ago when my eighty-three-year-old father had an abdominal aortic aneurysm that required repair. I didn't think my father would survive the recommended "open" procedure and so I searched for a cutting-edge vascular surgeon who could fix his problem less invasively with a stent. Dr. George Fielding sent us to see his colleague, Dr. Cayne. Dad went back to work a week after Dr. Cayne's surgery, and as I write this he has just celebrated his eighty-sixth birthday!

Becoming a Breast Surgeon

Susan M. Love, MD, FACS

PEOPLE OFTEN ASK ME how I became a breast surgeon. I always suspect that they want me to say that my mother died of breast cancer (she did not) or something similarly heart-wrenching. In fact, I became a breast surgeon because at the time it was my only choice.

I applied to medical school when there were still quotas as to how many women a program would accept— 5 percent at most schools. My premed adviser told me that I should not go to medical school, because I would be taking some boy's place who would consequently be drafted and die in Vietnam. I persisted, nonetheless, and as I started my third year of medical school, a law called Title

IX was passed, stating that all schools receiving government money were prohibited from discriminating against
women. The professional schools were the first to drop
their quotas, and the class went from 10 percent women
to 30 percent in one year.

At the time, I thought I would be a cardiologist. I
thought the motto "Send your broken heart to Dr. Love"
was too good to pass up. But in the third year, when we
rotated on all the specialties, it was clear that surgery was the
only one I liked. I especially enjoyed the immediacy of it.
You could see someone in the emergency room and suspect
that he had appendicitis, and then take him to the operating
room and find out if it was true. And you could cure people.
As opposed to internal medicine, where you treat chronic
diseases, in surgery when you take someone's appendix out,
that person can never get appendicitis again! Cured! It was
clear-cut (pun intended). It is ironic that I ended up a breast
cancer surgeon, in a field where surgery is not always cura-
tive and the disease is anything but clear-cut.

My applying to a surgical training program brought
the sexism out in full force. One well-known program in
New York asked me what kind of birth control I used, while
a prominent Boston program asked me how I would be
able to get close enough to a patient to operate when I was
pregnant. I told them that even pregnant, my belly would
be smaller than that of many of their current surgeons, a
comment which did not endear me to the interviewers.

I trained at Beth Israel Hospital in Boston, which was
more supportive than most. Even so, I was only the second

woman to finish the general surgery program and the first woman on the staff in general surgery.

I went into private practice in 1979. At that time I was adamant that I did not want to be a breast surgeon, because in those days the only ones who did breast surgery were surgeons that either were retiring or were not good enough for "real surgery." "I can do big operations just as well as the next guy," I was heard to proclaim at the time. Little did I know where things were headed.

What I found was that the patients other doctors were willing to send to me were all women with breast problems. I think they were afraid to send me men or thought that it was inappropriate. The women, however, were starving for information about what was happening and why. I quickly found that I could make a much bigger difference to a woman with breast cancer than to a man with a hernia. It was the early days of breast conservation surgery for cancer. Good studies from Italy showed that lumpectomy and radiation were just as effective as mastectomy for most women. Yet American surgeons continued to suggest that it was true only for Italian women with Italian breast cancer, and would never work on American women with American breast cancer. As I saw more and more of these women, what started out as a career *became a mission*. Hard as it is to believe today, there were no surgeons who specialized in breast cancer in those days. In fact, one chief of surgery warned me that I would never be able to make a living as a breast surgeon. Years later, I laugh at that prediction every time the American Association of Breast Surgeons has their annual meeting!

My life as a breast surgeon has taught me many lessons. It was humbling to recognize the responsibility and trust I had been given. For patients to allow you to operate on them, the ultimate intimate act, they must decide that you are worthy and, in fact, wonderful. Some surgeons, over time, start believing their own press—that they *are* that wonderful. It is critical for a surgeon to acknowledge that she or he is human and far from a god.

To keep my own psyche in check, I had a ritual I would go through with every operation. I made sure I was in the operating room while the patient was still awake, and I held her hand as she went to sleep. This is the scariest time for a patient, and I was the only one in the room whom she knew. My presence calmed the patient but also served to remind me of the enormous trust that had been given to me to do my very best for her. Once she was asleep, I would go out and scrub my hands, using that time to review the technical task that was ahead. When I returned to the room, the patient would be draped and only a square of flesh would be visible, all the better for me to focus on the disembodied breast and the cancer hiding within. Once the operation was over, the drapes would be removed and the patient would reemerge. I always made sure to talk to patients in the recovery room, completing the circle and reinforcing their personhood.

It is all too easy to sashay into the operating room when the patient is already draped, perform your technical task, and then not see the patient again until the next day. With that approach, I think that surgeons soon lose track of the fact that these are not disembodied organs but real people they are working on, people who deserve the very best. To not continually acknowledge that fact is what I consider the first of three common surgical sins.

Along with the responsibility and trust that patients bestow upon their surgeon is the obligation by the surgeon to educate patients so that they can make the best decisions. Too often, as surgeons, we figure out what we would do if we were the patient and then suggest that as the best option. In fact, we are *not* them and sometimes are not anything like them.

To believe that we always know what is best for another person is a second surgical sin. What I would do if I were diagnosed with breast cancer is dependent on my neuroses, my feelings about my body, my risk tolerance, and my relationship with my mother. It has nothing to do with what the patient should do. My job is to educate the patient as to what we know and what we don't know *and* then to explain to her the risks and help her to explore her own neuroses, her feelings about her body, her risk tolerance, and her relationship with her mother. I have often been surprised by a woman with a low-grade, easily removed tumor who tells me she wants both breasts off. It may be overkill from a medical point of view, but I did not sit at her mother's deathbed at the age of thirteen and can never know what scars and fears she was left with.

Then there are the women who are scared to death of

traditional treatments and who cannot bring themselves to undergo chemotherapy that might be lifesaving. Who am I to say what is best for another adult? My job is to listen, and to explain the options, and to help her decide what she wants to do rather than what I would do or think she should do. I have been known to suggest that the doctor who says, "If you were my wife" should be asked if he likes his wife!

The third surgical sin is to become disengaged. After ten years of telling women that they have breast cancer and discussing treatment options, it becomes all too easy to tune out and repeat your spiel by rote while thinking about what to cook for dinner. It is critical to see each patient as a person with parents and sometimes children. It is vital that surgeons get to know their patients well enough to see their disease in context and from their viewpoint. It is important to still be able to feel, acknowledge, and address their fear, even when it is unrealistic. When a patient becomes "the mastectomy in room 320," it is time to hang up your scalpel and find other work. I must admit that twenty years into my career as a breast surgeon, I started to notice my mind wandering as I talked to someone about her new cancer. Horrified, I realized that *even I* could get burned out. I reevaluated my life and decided that I needed to move from taking care of breast cancers one by one to tackling the whole problem. I left clinical practice to do research and try to eradicate breast cancer once and for all.

This decision is probably best explained by a story

about two women surgeons who were standing in a stream. Every ten minutes or so, a body would come floating down the stream and the women would catch it, resuscitate the person, and deliver her back safely to the shore. After a while one of the surgeons got out of the water and started to walk upstream. Her colleague yelled out to her, "Where are you going? These bodies keep on coming."

"I know," shouted back the first surgeon from the shore. "I am going to find out who is throwing them in!"

Being a surgeon is not something that you change or grow out of. It is part of who you are, your identity. Surgeons want to fix things! And being a breast cancer surgeon means you want to cut it out, not just the tumor but the whole disease. My quest to eradicate breast cancer defines why I became a breast surgeon.

Editor's Note: An inspiring surgeon, Dr. Sue Love was one of my teachers at Harvard's Beth Israel Hospital in Boston. She is one of the nation's leading experts on breast cancer and is the author of Dr. Love's Breast Book, *which soon will publish its 5th edition in seven languages. Dr. Love is among the first generation of dedicated breast surgeons.*

The Burn Unit

Arthur W. Perry, MD, FACS

Y OU NEVER FORGET that first burned patient. The charred skin, the hair frizzed from heat, and the smell. Burned human flesh has a distinct odor, different from beef or chicken. An odor that, once smelled, stays with you forever. As the dozens, then hundreds of burn victims that rolled through the emergency room door eventually became routine, I was continually reminded of the horror by reactions from the medley of medical students and surgical residents who spent a month on the service with me.

Perhaps the most respected place in a hospital is the burn unit. The agony that occurs inside those walls is overshadowed by the miracles that are performed there. A place where life and death play out on a daily basis, where pain is so common that intravenous morphine is served up like fries at McDonald's. Burn units are usually found in larger hospitals, often university teaching hospitals. They are so labor-intensive that scores of attending surgeons, residents in training, and medical students are needed to perform the daily rituals that combine lifesaving medical and surgical care.

When I was the burn fellow in the New York Hospital–Cornell Burn Center in the 1980s, my year seemed like a decade. I welcomed the opportunity, wedged between general surgery and plastic surgery residencies, to learn to take care of the sickest patients in the hospital. New York Hospital was just the place to do that. It was the busiest burn center in the United States: over 800 burned patients flowed through the doors during my year, a pace that rivaled military hospitals. The center, now named after William Randolph Hearst, today admits more than 1,300 patients each year.

Having just spent three years in general surgery at Harvard, I was up for any challenge. But the grueling every-other-night call schedule and the steady pace of critically ill patients allowed me to shed ten pounds of extra weight during my first month.

The fates of the twenty-eight intensive care unit patients and more than thirty "walking wounded" were arranged carefully on an infamous dry-erase board. While there was a steady flow of different names in and out of the unit, the patients seemed to remain the same. There was always a New York City fireman nursing third-degree burns on the kneecaps and thighs, just above where the fire-protective boots reached. There was the Orthodox Jewish infant whose shirt had become engulfed in flames from Sabbath candles. There was the homeless man, torched for sport by wiseguys under the 59th Street Bridge. And there were the AIDS patients, transferred from Sloan-Kettering after losing their skin in a disease called toxic epidermal necrolysis, a peculiar reaction to antibiotics.

But there were also burns that I could never forget. Like the twenty-eight-year-old man who fell into a vat of acid in a Queens factory and swam around until he was fished out by coworkers. With burns covering 100 percent of his body, sparing only his eyeballs, he was brought into my unit, talking normally, asking how long he'd have to be in the hospital. The doctors and nurses in the burn unit were somber, because we all knew that within a few days, this man would be dead. A 100 percent chemical burn is a lethal injury. Within a few hours the swelling would be so profound that his airway would be squeezed, causing respiratory distress. And so a breathing tube was placed, bridging the swollen upper airway, allowing oxygen to reach the lungs. But a physiologic nightmare was occurring before our eyes—a disturbance in the immune system so profound that infection couldn't be fought. By the forty-eight hour mark, the patient's systems began to fail—first the kidneys, then the lungs, and finally the heart. Death quickly followed.

While most burns at Cornell were industrial accidents, every few months the subway surfers would be carted in.

The urge to ride on top of New York City subway trains is one that most people can squelch. But given a dare and more than a few beers, the top of a subway car can become a vehicle for death. There's no burn that is preferred, but electrocution is one of the more vicious ways to die. The subway surfers whose skulls don't crack against low-lying beams but who do contact the 625 volts of the "third rail", or overlying electrical wires, buy an often-one-way ticket into the burn unit. When electrical current enters the body, it travels through tissues and eventually exits through the path of least resistance, finding a piece of nearby metal, leaving the body explosively, sometimes arcing through the air. Along the way, structures like bone and muscle heat up and and cook like soup in a crockpot.

Burn units don't usually see lightning strikes or third-rail victims: the electricity kills them instantly by causing a fatal irregular rhythm of the heart. But the patients who *do* survive suffer an agonizing fate, like the nineteen-year-old subway surfer I cared for. The electrical current had entered his hand, which fried like a mummy, and coursed through his body, hitting his heart before blasting out what looked like a shrapnel wound in his thigh. The current traveled along his muscles of the arm, swelling them and cutting off their blood supply. An immediate, painful fasciotomy, a procedure that sliced open the white connective tissue over each and every muscle in the arm, needed to be done to save his arm. After filleting the arm open, we bathed it in the nectar of the burn unit— the ubiquitous Silvadene antibacterial cream. By the next morning, the insidious nature of the electricity became obvious. In the operating room, the team used knives, scissors, and (paradoxically) electrocautery to pare down dead tissue. Trying to save as much of the arm as possible, we erred on the conservative side, leaving as much as we could. But by two days later, the progressive nature of an electrical injury reared its ugly head. Back in the OR, little of the arm had survived. And so the difficult decision to amputate the arm of this subway surfer, out for a little fun in a most reckless way, was made. This one lived, but his life would never be the same.

Some of the most challenging problems were presented by patients who had been trapped in smoke-filled buildings. The toxins in smoke cause rapid swelling of the airway. Combined with tissue billowing from burns around the mouth, the airway can quickly close off, suffocating the victim. By the time patients hit the emergency room, the airway near their vocal cords can be reduced from the diameter of a pinball to the size of a pea. Without an emergency breathing tube, death comes quickly from asphyxiation. My job was to inspect the airway with a device called a bronchoscope, which looks like a mini-colonoscope, a tube with a lens on the end of it. The tube is passed through the nose with the patient awake, with every passing second resulting in even more swelling. Through the bloated tissue, the target—the vocal cords—comes into view. There's a certain amount of sport to performing a bronchoscopy. To win this game, the tube must be passed through the paired cords, which act like a goalie protecting the net, keeping bread crumbs, raisins, and now the bronchoscope out of the lungs. But after hundreds of these bronchoscopies, I would never be denied the victory of popping a breathing tube through the cords and down the trachea. Once the scope is through the cords, a lifesaving endotracheal tube slides over the scope, bringing oxygen to the lungs.

I'd come home from a day's work with a giant red stain on my belly and one on each thigh. This was blood that had soaked through both my sterile surgical gown and my scrubs. Burn cases are bloody cases. Each night I'd shower, watching the dried blood swirl down the drain. And each night I'd be thankful for the hepatitis B experimental vaccine I'd taken during my surgical residency at Harvard, because that deadly virus has been known to penetrate intact skin.

In essence, burn care is a race. Cut off the dead, burned skin and fat before the bacteria eat it. Bacteria love dead tissue, and humans live in a delicate balance with legions of bacteria. In fact, without bacteria in our intestines we become vitamin K–deficient and our blood can't clot properly. Even physicians don't realize that bacteria are needed for proper wound healing. Animals that live in germ-free environments heal poorly. But in a burned patient, the bacterial balance is skewed in favor of the bugs. Despite intravenous antibiotics and virtually bathing in Silvadene, patients with large burns are nearly always invaded by infection.

So the team of an attending, a burn fellow, and two surgical residents, an anesthesiologist and her resident, three nurses, and a medical student or two gather in the operating room as soon as the patient's vital signs stabilize, to cheese-slice through the charred tissue, causing furious bleeding that challenges the skills of the best anesthesiologists. Ten pints of blood are typically lost in these cases, pouring out of the wounds, onto the drapes, into piles of gauze, and onto the floor. As I slice through the burned tissue, I tell the anesthesiologist to give the patient a couple more units of blood. The nurse wipes sweat off my brow, as the operating room temperature of 90 degrees contributes to my fatigue. Patients without skin lose body heat rapidly, and the first sign of hypothermia can be cardiac arrest. So the scene is set—a furious pace of a team of surgeons, some slicing off charred tissue, others harvesting skin from unburned "donor" areas, and still others stretching out the skin with a mechanical *mesher*, which expands the skin an additional 50 percent. Still others apply the skin grafts to the burned areas, stapling it in place and immobilizing the areas with gauze and plaster splints. A buzz of activity is taking place in a tropical atmosphere. No more than 20 percent of the body surface area can be operated on, because the insult is too great for the body, so the patient is sent back to the burn unit to heal and recover, only to repeat the ritual over and over, until the last dime-sized piece of burned skin is healed. Only then will the months and years of rehabilitation—both physical and psychological—begin.

No time for food on surgery days, but I might grab one of the high-calorie, high-protein drinks that populate the refrigerators in the recovery room. By the time we wheel the patient back to the unit, the next patient is already in the OR, being readied for an identical procedure. Different burn, different limb, another ten pints of blood, poured in the vein, leaking out the wound. Three days a week, eight hours a day. Acres and acres of skin grafted in thousands of procedures.

When not in the operating room, I'm running the care of the most critically ill patients in the hospital. Patients with fluid needs that shift by the hour, depending on what phase of the burn they are in. Patients who have developed sepsis, bacteria in their blood, causing problems with their hearts, kidneys, and lungs. And yes, running the codes. Those are the cardiac arrests. Hardly a day goes by without a death in that high-volume unit. Deaths affect every doctor and nurse in the unit. We rationalize the deaths by citing statistics. A seventy-year-old with a 70 percent burn has less than a 5 percent chance of survival. And so the die is cast at the time of the burn, though the staff would give 100 percent to make that one person the 5 percent that would live. But as with the acid swimmer, we had a pretty good idea of who would die when they came through the door. The ones that hurt us were the unexpected deaths. The twenty-year-old with the 60 percent burn who had a one-in-three chance of dying—we wouldn't let him die.

And every now and then a personal acquaintance wound up as my patient. Because I had eaten at Ben's Chinese restaurant in upstate New York, it was a comfort to Ben's hot oil-burned brother-in-law when he learned that I was a fan of his General Tso's chicken. While burns to the hands are not life-threatening, they can limit function and render a person unemployable. Thankfully, after surgery and therapy, the hands healed and were functional, albeit scarred.

By the end of the year, I had a love-hate relationship with burns. As a typical cocky surgeon, I knew there was no one better at burn care, but the daily stress of constantly dealing with life-and-death situations was grinding, and I was ready to move on to my plastic surgery residency. While I now operate on aged faces and large noses, I recently became affiliated with the Cornell/Columbia plastic surgery residency program. Twenty-three years after leaving the burn unit, I now attend monthly plastic surgery conferences in the very same room where I once helped save the lives of hundreds of burn victims.

Doc's Lessons

A. John Popp, MD, FACS

THE YEAR WAS 1977. It was early morning, and I had just begun to evaluate my first patient. My administrative assistant was usually busy during this time doing other things; seeing her this morning immediately signaled to me that something out of the ordinary was going on.

"There is someone on the phone named Doc Willard. When I explained that you were busy seeing patients, he said you'd take his call," she said.

There was no hesitation on my part. Dr. Charles Willard—he and everyone else preferred "Doc"—was an icon in my little hometown in western New York, about an hour east of Buffalo. That's where I had spent my first seventeen years. Hearing his name triggered images and memories of my childhood. I remembered an unsorted amalgamation of factual data, wishful thinking, and rumors, all gathered from uncorroborated boyhood memories.

Doc grew up on a farm but, unlike many in our community, where sons worked on their father's farms until they bought their own, he aspired to become a physician. George Turner, the wealthiest man in town and reputed to be a "real" millionaire—at that time no small accomplishment—struck a deal with Willard during the depths of the Depression. Turner would pay for medical school at Cornell if Willard would return to be the town doctor.

Over the years a few other doctors came to town, but Doc Willard was the busiest. He was my family's doctor and brought me into the world. And it seemed that my most traumatic times were spent in his office, where his calm demeanor quelled my fears. I recall injuring my right index finger in a school accident. The bleeding and pain were so intense that I thought my finger had been nearly severed. I was just six years old, but I recall walking the five blocks to Doc's office holding the finger in place so it could be reattached. Once the sutures were in place and Doc had reassured me, it was back to business as usual. Decades later, as I look at the small white scar, the aftermath of that injury, I am struck by how insignificant it looks. Time sure does heal wounds.

Doc Willard played a recurring role in my life, leading right up to my acceptance into medical school. With my acceptance letter in hand, I accompanied my mother to Doc's office for a routine visit. He told my mother that he would no longer be charging me for medical care, now that I was a colleague in the medical profession! He said that was how professionals treated each other. Thereafter, when we met occasionally, he would greet me as a colleague and inquire about my ongoing medical education.

In high school it had become a secret dream of mine to finish medical school and return and join Doc in practice. Those inchoate dreams changed rapidly when I entered medical school, discovered an aptitude for anatomy, and began thinking about applied anatomy and the field of surgery as a career choice. It was cemented by my study of neuroanatomy the next semester, as I developed a fascination with the complex circuitry involved in the nervous system. This nascent interest was further heightened when I observed the logical approach that neurosurgeons used to treat patients with disorders of the brain and spine. I felt electrified by this discovery, and my interest continues to this day.

And so it was to be neurosurgery, known both in puns and in surgical circles as the most "cerebral" of the surgical specialties. Once that decision was made, I put in twelve years of training to become a neurosurgeon.

During those years of training and my early years in clinical practice, I rarely saw Doc. When I did, our interactions were always cordial and ones in which we shared a common bond. But Doc Willard never called. So when the phone rang and it was Doc calling, I knew at once that it was on a matter of great significance.

I was aroused from these reminiscences when Doc said, "Aida's in a coma."

For the layperson, the term *coma* might simply mean someone is unconscious. But for neurosurgeons, the term gets our attention, since the sudden onset of coma often mandates rapid treatment. In short order, the possible causes of coma run through our minds, and before another sentence is uttered, treatment options are being considered. With urgency in my voice I asked what the cause of the coma was and how long Aida, Doc's wife, had been in a coma.

"About two years." He went on, "We have full-time nurses, but it is getting more difficult each day, and I really don't want to put her into a nursing home. You know how that will end. Aida was operated on in Rochester by 'the best.' She had hydrocephalus, John, but they don't know the cause. She had two shunting procedures to drain the fluid, but they didn't work. I don't want to bother you, but would you give me your opinion?" Then as an afterthought he added, "There is no rush."

Hydrocephalus is also known as water on the brain. Each second, twenty-four hours a day, the brain produces one-fifteenth of a teaspoon of clear cerebrospinal fluid (CSF); that's nearly a pint a day. CSF is produced in the spaces of the brain called ventricles and flows through a complicated series of channels. It travels around the surface of the brain and is reabsorbed into the blood at the top of the head. Any blockage of this circulation from a brain abnormality, such as a tumor or even certain birth defects, can cause a rapid buildup of fluid. That results in pressure on the brain. And as when a slowly moving stream is dammed, the water will back up. The resulting disorder, hydrocephalus, can lead to coma and death.

By coincidence, I had already scheduled my semiannual trip back to my boyhood home for two days later. When I arrived at Doc and Aida's home, all her medical records were available. When I stimulated her arms and legs, she responded normally. However, she would not open her eyes. The x-rays were less sophisticated than what we have today. There was no CT scan—not surprising, because when Aida had first developed her neurological problem many hospitals in the United States did not have CT scanners. This invention had revolutionized the quality and precision of neurosurgical patient care and had earned its inventor, Godfrey Hounsfield, a Nobel Prize in 1979.

A plain x-ray series of Aida's skull was normal, but a special procedure called a *ventriculogram* was most revealing. By 1977, the year I saw Aida, that procedure was outmoded; CT scans had rendered it obsolete several years earlier. Ventriculograms were complicated and required air to be injected into the ventricles of the brain to aid in the diagnosis of the cause of the hydrocephalus. While this procedure now seems hopelessly primitive by today's standards, it was often the best we had before the arrival of the CT scan. Aida had had no diagnostic studies after the ventriculogram, and after two operations designed to reduce the pressure in the brain did not help, her doctors, including her doctor husband, had said, "Enough."

After carefully reviewing her x-rays and her history, I felt that I could not precisely determine the exact cause of Aida's decline. However, my review of the primitive ventriculogram suggested a small suspicious area at the back of the brain that could be the culprit. I advised obtaining a CT scan. I told Doc that it could be done at the closest CT scanner, in Rochester, a one-hour drive from their home. Without hesitation Doc decided that he wanted Aida to come to my hospital in Albany, an ambulance trip of four and a half hours.

Within a week Aida Willard, age sixty-nine, was admitted to the Albany Medical Center, where I was a young neurosurgeon. The CT scan confirmed my suspicion. Aida had a very small but critically placed, unusual collection of blood vessels in her brain that caused a buildup of the fluid. Given the location of the problem and her general condition, surgical removal of the abnormality was not a good option. After a long discussion with Doc, we decided to place a new type of shunt, hoping for the best but knowing this approach, already tried twice, might not work a third time. For Doc, who had been practicing medicine for over forty years, it was a difficult decision, a very personal decision involving both his love for his wife and his knowledge of the complex medical issues involved. When Doc and I met early in the morning before surgery, we were both weary. Doc had slept poorly, worrying about his wife, but was hopeful that surgery would help her; I had spent the night, as I often do with perplexing cases, sleeping fitfully as my subconscious tries to make sense of the confounding data of the patient who will be undergoing surgery the next day.

Surgery lasted only forty-five minutes; I inserted a shunt that drained spinal fluid from the cavities of the brain through a silicon tube that channeled under the skin, ending up in the abdomen, where the fluid was reabsorbed. During surgery I had carefully measured the pressure in the brain and found it to be increased—a sign that the prior shunts were not working.

Aida's response to surgery was nothing short of miraculous. Within a day she began to respond; soon she was looking around, and a few days later she began to speak. If life has paybacks, I think Doc earned this one for being my role model. He was grateful beyond words.

Years later, I visited Doc and Aida on one of my trips home. Aida was sitting at the table conversing normally. I learned that she was playing bridge again—a former passion. She was troubled by a desire to remember what happened to her during those years of coma. I reminded her gently the lack of memory was nature's way of protecting her from bad memories, and that memories of those lost years would never return to her.

Aida lived another seven years and died from an unrelated illness. I occasionally saw Aida again, and Doc was always happy to tell others in my hometown about my diagnostic and surgical prowess. Despite being the recipient of such praise, I felt lucky to have been Aida's last neurosurgeon rather than her first!

About twenty years after Aida's operation, I received another phone call from Doc. "John, the doctors tell me that I have a brain tumor and need surgery. I would like to come to see you for a second opinion."

When I saw Doc, he had aged—no surprise, since he was nearly ninety at the time. I thought of his wife's primitive x-rays as I ordered an MRI of his brain. This sophisticated scan, a successor to CT scans, showed a large meningioma, a type of benign tumor, in a difficult location. Removal of these slowly growing tumors often requires long and complex operations. Doc was nearly asymptomatic except for vague headaches. Decisions about when to perform surgery are never easy, but a surgeon's decision-making process includes balancing the risks and benefits of surgery. It is often easier to make the decision to operate than to not operate, because action is valued more than *in*action, particularly among surgeons.

Before me was a beloved individual, a colleague, a role model, and an icon to his community and to me. But he was also a patient who was nearly ninety and virtually asymptomatic; and one who, if we decided to proceed with surgery, would be exposed to the serious risks in a long, complicated operation. I felt that the cost of achieving a cure was too great. When I told him so, he only said, *"Primum non nocere"* (First do no harm) —a fundamental element of the physician's credo dating from the time of Hippocrates.

Doc's family contacted me several weeks after his discharge from the hospital. He had died unexpectedly in his sleep, most likely from heart disease.

As I write this, I reflect on the powerful influence Doc Willard had on the gestation and development of my career in medicine. Physicians now practice in an environment that has changed dramatically from the one in which Doc practiced and both he and his wife were patients. In this "managed care" era, some physicians have been accused of being too commercial, making too many errors, and having unsavory ties with industry. However, I know many physicians who serve as powerful role models and possess an enduring sense of obligation to their patients, community, and profession. As surgeons they understand their responsibility not only to perform operations but also to provide thoughtful counsel, even when surgery may not be indicated. As an educator of future neurosurgeons in this complex practice environment, I believe that the moral compass for practicing with integrity is an unimpeachable commitment to the tenets of professionalism that for me was first demonstrated by Doc Willard.

Editor's Note: As a medical student, I vividly remember Dr. Popp's neurosurgery lectures, which helped shape my surgical career. Now a Harvard neurosurgeon, he spent much of his career as Chairman of Surgery at the Albany Medical College.

DANIEL

Meghann Kaiser, MD

AROUND TWO OR THREE in the morning, my medical students gather around me. As resident, I buy them each a cup of vending-machine coffee and a shrink-wrapped pastry, and together we huddle in the call room and pretend we are at some macabre slumber party and not on trauma call, waiting for the other shoe to drop. Those who do not doze off start asking me questions. For the most part the questions are typical enough: why pick surgery, what was the grossest thing you've ever seen, and so on. But occasionally a more introspective pupil digs up something more challenging. How do you live with it? How do you live with the mistakes you've made?

This is a fair question, but one without a satisfying answer that I know of. I am a human, which means I make mistakes. But I am also a surgeon, which means that I am not the only one who pays dearly for those mistakes, sometimes indefinitely. Even with this burden, however, we must find some way to keep going. I am certainly not suggesting that we discard it at the side of the road, but rather that we bundle it up into a manageable pack that we carry between the shoulder blades, where the weight may slow us down a bit but not stop us entirely.

I glance at my little apprentices slumped against the wall, like horses dozing off while standing. In the pause after I trail off and just before the trauma pager beeps again, I inevitably think of Daniel, whether I want to or not. He is not part of the stories I tell them; why would he be? There's no sense to be made of his story—no lesson to be learned or moral to be had. Only the heaviness.

Daniel's parents conceived him in their mid-forties, after ten childless years. He was everything a miracle baby should be: curious but soft-spoken, playful, trusting, gentle, and strangely wistful. He played the violin with a thoughtful intent his nine years couldn't account for, and played soccer with the reckless enthusiasm only a child can muster. I never knew this Daniel. When they brought him into the trauma bay, he was limp and not breathing.

The red welt of a seat belt across his chest bore witness both to the immense love and to the tragedy that fate had allotted him. But his heart was undeterred and his pupils reactive to light: with those signs, physicians know that there is still hope. A crew of doctors and nurses stabilized him and rushed him to the CT scanner. I had hoped to find bleeding in the brain that might account for his findings—a devastating injury certainly, but potentially reversible. I hovered over the computer screen, digesting the images as fast as the scanner could obtain them. There was generalized swelling of the brain but nothing resembling the discrete bleeding I wanted to see. I turned away, deflated.

For the next half-hour I busied myself finding Daniel a bed in the pediatric ICU, called a neurosurgery consult, and placed intravenous lines. That was when the page came from the radiologist, who by then had had the chance to review the scans herself. It was, I remember her saying, the strangest and most chilling picture she had ever seen: the skull had jumped forward—and entirely off—the spine, crushing the tail end of his brain stem. The spinal cord had separated from the brain. He was, in effect, internally decapitated.

What followed this revelation was sheer chaos. Pediatricians, neurosurgeons, orthopedic surgeons, and trauma surgeons like myself all swarmed the bed. Trauma presents a curious social challenge, in that young, previously healthy people are frequently affected, forcing families to face life-altering decisions for which they are wholly unprepared. It may take several days for them to make peace with the unforgiving inevitable; and in the meantime, for better or worse, we doctors sometimes forge ahead with a retrospectively hopeless course of treatment. It is, admittedly, much more for the family than for the patient, but in the midst of such cruelty, a few extra days with their loved one is a mercy we can and should provide. Daniel's father was already at the bedside with a small flock of church friends surrounding him. Daniel's mother held her son's hand. I told them the matter was very grave and that Daniel's brain had been severely affected, but that was all. I consoled them—and myself—with the assurance that he was not suffering.

Somewhere in the night, things began to deteriorate. His blood pressure became unstable and his pupils less reactive. His mother, sensing the agitation of the nurses, knew the situation had worsened. She pleaded with me in staggering desperation: do something, do everything, do whatever needs to be done. And I was faced with a choice—intervene with an invasive and potentially painful procedure that would do the patient no good; or tell his parents, right then and there, that the son they had driven home from a pizza party just ten hours earlier would not live through the night. It was too soon for any of us. I summoned the neurosurgeon back to the bedside, where a drain was placed to relieve the pressure in Daniel's skull. His vitals stabilized. He would live through the night.

In the coming days, I gathered Daniel's parents and extended family together with multiple specialists, all saying the same thing: Daniel, as you knew him, is gone. There is nothing left now but a few physiologic processes that cannot even sustain life on their own. Either withdraw care or he will succumb to infection in the coming months; but either way, he will never come back. It was a gently delivered but necessarily harsh onslaught of truth.

There were outbursts, tears, prayers, and at last, acceptance. As a matter of professionalism, we always had these discussions in a separate room out of Daniel's presence, although we knew he couldn't hear us.

Daniel's parents made plans to take him off life support early the following week. More family flew in, and funeral arrangements were made. But when his mother stood up to leave his side that last night, a tiny tear formed in the corner of his eye. I took it to mean a reflex; she took it to mean a miracle. The nurse applied eyedrops, but the tears continued to collect and fall. I took a flashlight to the bedside and began to examine him. There were no corneal abrasions or other injuries that I could see. But when I straightened up and paused to regard him from afar, I suddenly realized that he was watching me. *And he was crying.*

For a brief moment I was no different from his mother—overjoyed, amazed, senseless with awe. I paged my attending, the neurosurgeon, and anyone else I could think of. Then, in the midst of my jubilation, it occurred to me that Daniel still had not moved. Not his legs, not his arms, not even his face; only his eyes, darting back and forth in sheer terror. By the time the neurosurgeon returned my call, an empty tinge of horror in his voice, I had already put two and two together. Daniel was "locked in." We hear about it occasionally with adults: a stroke affecting the brainstem leaves its victim able to communicate only through movements of the eyes. Daniel's injury had affected the same nerve cells. So now, although he could still hear, see, feel, and know his world, this nine-year-old boy was no longer a part of it.

He stayed in the ICU for a few weeks after that. His mother didn't leave his side. Child psychologists migrated in and out, trying to explain to him the unexplainable, and each time his response was the same: just a slow, steady tear fall. Eventually he was transferred to a nursing home, where his ventilator and a myriad of other needs could be closely managed. But I think about him daily. That night, in my weak desire to spare his parents—and myself—the sudden shock of his loss, did I unknowingly condemn this innocent child to a lifetime of hell? Did I make the right choice? Was it ever my choice to make? Was it anyone's? If only I, they, and he had known—and really understood—but can we ever really understand? What if life isn't always life?

My trauma pager goes off, awakening me from this recurring nightmare, summoning me to the needs of yet another critically ill patient. Daniel is always in my thoughts, and for a moment I am still, trapped with him, unable to move, breathe, speak, or escape. Then come the sounds of my medical student from the bunk above, as her feet drop to the floor with a thud and she heads for the light switch. The harsh, fluorescent light of 4 A.M. flashes across the room, and I grant for myself what I could not for Daniel: I unlock and open the door, and I am gone.

Editors's Note: Dr. Kaiser's story reveals a side of surgeons the public doesn't see. Dealing with this injury shows the torment that physicians feel when their patients have a poor outcome. This story perhaps truly describes a fate worse than death and the continued memory of a doctor who wrestles with her decisions for years.

A Shot for the Pain

Ian Dorward, MD

Tony Martin shot himself in the head. He held a .22-caliber handgun to his right temple and pulled the trigger, but at an angle such that the bullet came out the middle of his forehead. His wife found him walking from the couch to the refrigerator and back again, mumbling in semi-words and bleeding down his shirt.

Paramedics had intubated Tony in the back of an ambulance and rushed him here, so that I, as the senior resident member of the neurosurgery team, could help take care of him. When I first walked into the room, a nurse who was hunched over the bed yelled, "Thank God, he's here!" I thought she was making fun of me at first—some play on neurosurgeons and their egos. But no, it turns out she really thought I could help.

"Look at this!" she yelled, turning her head over her shoulder to see me better. In her hands she held two gauze sponges that she pressed firmly to his right temple and his forehead. "He's got gray stuff coming out!"

"You know what that is, right?" I asked.

She puzzled over the question, not sure whether or not it was rhetorical.

"You should let it come out," I said, reaching toward her with a calming gesture. "It's like a pop-off valve. Let it go."

She backed away, standing beside the bed and staring at his head. She still clutched the bloody gauze sponges.

I squeezed into some latex gloves and approached the head of the bed to examine him. He opened his eyes to my voice, looked around, and tried to reach for his endotracheal tube. His eyes still reacted to light, and his other cranial nerves all functioned properly. I tried talking to him—"Tony, squeeze my hand"—but his thoughts, had he any at all, were elsewhere.

"Tony, don't worry, we'll get you through this," I said, doubting that he heard me.

As I began to strip off one of my latex gloves, I noticed the nurse still staring, transfixed, at his forehead. A little core of brain had risen there, like gray goo extruded by a Play-Doh Fun Factory.

"Can I have one of those?" I said to the nurse.

"What?"

"One of those gauzes in your hands."

She looked at one and slowly stretched it toward me,

as if it were incriminating evidence she was forced to relinquish. I grabbed it with my one still-gloved hand and swiped the brain off Tony's forehead, then handed it back to her. She stared at it, a smear of his frontal lobe in the palm of her hand.

I called the operating room, the anesthesia team, and the attending neurosurgeon. A strange sense of calm settled into my voice; somehow I knew we would be able to help this guy. While waiting several minutes for the OR nurses to ready the room for us, I sought out the patient's wife.

She had been sequestered in a windowless room the size of a modest kitchen pantry. A social worker met me at the room's door and whispered something about an episode of screaming and crying and falling to the floor, just so I would know. I stepped in and sat down beside her on a green leather chair. As I introduced myself, she remained composed long enough to tell me her name—Sarah—before shrieking and clutching at her head. I placed my hand gently on her shoulder and waited.

She shuddered for a moment, then came around all at once. With an abrupt turn she looked straight into my eyes—tear-soaked hair dangling into her face—and grasped my forearm, letting her nails dig in.

"You have to help him. You have to make this go away. You have to *fix* him."

I looked at her eyes for a moment—deep blue and burning, like a blazing oil slick on the open ocean—and replied in the calmest voice I could muster.

"We intend to do everything we can to help him, Ms. Martin. He's very sick, as you know, but I think we have a good shot of getting him through this."

She shook her head violently and grabbed her hair. "Get him through this like he'll be alive or barely alive and sucking yogurt through a straw, or get him through this like he used to be? Get him through this as my Tony?"

This is the tricky part. Setting expectations. In that instant I had more power than I'll ever have wielding a scalpel. Hope is more delicate than brain. I played it safe, the cagey gambit to keep all doors open.

"It's just too early to say, Ms. Martin. This is a life-threatening injury, and he could die. But there's a decent chance that he could end up being very nearly like he used to be."

"Very nearly?" she repeated, scowling. "*Very nearly*? Is that all you can give me?"

Turns out that was all I could give her, because it was all I had.

The operation couldn't have gone better. We removed the frontal bones on both sides, nearly in their entirety. Then we opened up the dura, the thick layer surrounding the brain, and sewed in grafts—a couple of large pieces of tissue made from the sac from around a cow's heart, processed and sterilized—to make a nice roomy compartment for the injured and swollen brain. The whole right frontal lobe was "bombed out and depleted" as I once heard a neurosurgeon say: it was a heterogeneous mix of purples and yellows and grays, looking stomped-on or viciously stirred.

The bullet's entry and exit sites into the bone came out with the rest of the frontal skull. At the right temporal area, a stellate (star-shaped) pattern marked the point-blank impact; in the mid-forehead, the bone had exploded outward in multiple shards. Had someone else shot him, this bone would all be evidence; as it was, this bone was all trash. We pitched it in a red biohazard bag, where it knocked around with disposable suctions, drapes, and canisters of blood.

We obtained a CT scan of his head after the surgery, before taking him up to the intensive care unit. His was an unusual CT: the skull, which normally forms a stark, bright rim around the entire brain, looked like an open-topped vase or chalice into which Tony's essence had been poured.

Next we rolled him to the ICU, where his wife waited. As we pushed his bed up to the front entrance, she looked up at us but did not approach; instead, she paced back and forth in front of a row of empty chairs, her worrying assisted by something small and shiny that she held in her hand. Her mouth spoke words I couldn't hear.

When I checked on him later in the afternoon, he looked up at me and tried to talk around his breathing tube. He followed commands and moved all of his extremities with full strength. He would do fine.

"Will he be sad anymore?" his wife asked. "Like he was before?"

In the days that followed, Tony made great strides. The day after surgery we took out his breathing tube, and he started speaking rather normally. We fitted him with a little blue protective helmet so that he wouldn't inadvertently "brain" himself on a bed rail. Soon he moved out of the ICU and to the regular patient care floor, where his new personality quirks began to manifest themselves.

Tony, it seems, couldn't hold still. He would fidget on the edge of his bed, then hop up and walk to the bathroom mirror for a quick inspection of the long wound arcing from ear to ear along his scalp. Then he would turn around and pace back and forth in the room. After that, perhaps, a trip to the window to look out at the wind whipping through the trees in the park outside the hospital. Then back to the bed, for some more fidgeting, followed by another trip to the mirror. Things continued this way throughout the day.

His wife grew increasingly ecstatic as days went on. "You guys did it, you really saved him. He's a brand-new guy." They got caught making out in the bed, with Tony's roommate snoring gently six feet away from them. The next day they got caught again. They became inseparable, Sarah following Tony wherever his restless legs might take him. Within days he was doing well enough to be transferred to a rehabilitation hospital, where therapists could work with him several hours a day to rebuild his cognition and his strength—and where he and his wife could have a bit more privacy.

The next time I saw Tony was in our resident clinic, where we care for our multitude of uninsured patients. He had lost his job, of course, after he sustained a bullet to the brain, and his health insurance had vanished with it. I was glad, though, that I had the chance to see him again.

Unfortunately, Tony had developed a bit of a fluid collection beneath his wound. It happens sometimes that fluid from the healing tissues resorbs more slowly than it is made, leading to a swollen pocket of fluid under the scalp. In his case this had apparently increased in size quite gradually, such that his wife had barely even noticed it: "It was like one day I just opened my eyes and realized that, *poof*, his forehead had gotten huge."

His forehead had, indeed, gotten huge. So much fluid had built up that his skin sagged forward, hanging down over his brow ridge and almost obscuring his vision. The fluid swung back and forth when he walked—left foot, right foot, slosh, slosh, slosh. Worse, he had developed the habit of pressing on one side of his head to feel the wave roll across his brain and back again.

"Please don't do that," I told him the first time I saw this little trick. "There's nothing under there to protect your brain from your hand."

He nodded his head, said, "Yeah, okay," then promptly reached up and did it again.

The real problem with this fluid collection, though, was that it could be a harbinger of an infection. So after talking with the attending surgeon who had taken care of Tony before, we decided to admit him back to the hospital and drain and culture the fluid.

Tony and Sarah took the news rather well, excited as they were to have the fluid removed.

"I'll just be glad when we can fit him back into his helmet again," Sarah said.

Tony nodded and, to demonstrate the conundrum, tried to squeeze the thing back onto his head. The redundant scalp tissue mushroomed out the sides as he pressed the helmet on.

"Don't do that!" I almost shouted, reaching out to stay his hands. "I get it, I get it. It doesn't fit."

After cleaning a little patch of skin, I inserted a butterfly needle and began withdrawing. I started with the largest syringe the hospital had; I had brought eight with me. The yellow-tinged, clear fluid came out easily. Within seconds I had filled the first syringe, and I laid it on a bedside table and affixed another one to the needle. Tony watched me intently, wrenching his eyes all the way to the left as if trying to peer around his eye sockets at my hands. "That feels weird," he said. His wife left the room.

Several minutes later I moved on to my final syringe. I had made progress, there was no question, but the skin still bulged atop the remaining fluid. I had Tony hit the call button. A nurse came in within seconds. "Can you bring in more of these?" I asked.

She looked wide-eyed at the stack of full syringes, like loaded artillery shells, lying beside me on the table. "How many you need?"

"Better make it six more." I finally called it quits after removing over a pint. It wasn't until the last syringe that the scalp sank down fully, hugging the brain beneath and revealing the topography of hills and valleys of the brain.

I removed the needle and put a little Band-Aid over the hole.

Tony wasted no time in hopping out of bed and going to the bathroom mirror. I followed him. He scowled at his forehead, scrutinizing the new landscape up there. The right frontal lobe, where the bullet had passed, looked shriveled and small with respect to its counterpart. Tony reached up with his hand and gave it a little shove.

"Please, please don't do that," I begged. "That's your exposed brain. You don't want to damage your brain, do you?"

Tony smiled a little. "It's okay. I only touch the right side."

"But still, Tony, that's your brain," I began.

"No, really, it's okay. That was the sad part of me. I don't need it anymore. I got rid of it."

He turned squarely toward me. It took me a moment to realize that he wanted me to move out of his way, and I sheepishly stepped aside. He walked around the corner and out the door.

After saving some of the fluid to send to the lab and then cleaning up the considerable mess I had created, I walked out of the still-empty room. In the hallway, beside the door, Tony stood with his wife.

"Don't ever leave me again," she said to him, her hands locked in his.

"I won't," he said. "I promise. I'm fixed now." They kissed.

Editor's Note: Neurosurgeons operate on the organ that determines who we really are. You might say they operate on the personality and essence of being.

More Than Technique

William Silen, MD, FACS

IT MAY BE surprising to many to learn that the quality of a surgeon is defined only in small part by his or her technical expertise and finesse. It is a broadly held view, not only by laypersons but also by many physicians, that the slickest and quickest surgeon is the one you wish to be *your* surgeon. Recent advances in technology and the advent of novel procedures such as laparoscopic and thoracoscopic operations, as well as minimally invasive operations using tiny incisions in the neck and elsewhere, have only increased attention and interest in the manipulative skills of the surgeon. But while excellent technique is important in any successful surgical procedure, it is certainly not the only factor.

The most adverse results encountered in a surgical practice stem from either errors in diagnosis or errors in judgment. Such mistakes can be averted only by a surgeon who possesses a broad knowledge of medicine, and who leaves no stone unturned in carefully evaluating the results of laboratory tests, fancy new radiologic techniques (such as CT, MRI) and (2nd PET scans), and the suggestions of consulting colleagues in internal medicine and radiology. Improvement in diagnosis and judgment comes not only from continual assessment of a prescribed course of action in every case, but also from a willingness to confront and admit errors. As a teacher of medical students and residents, I am asked to review and critique many cases. From this experience, I offer two examples in which a more thoughtful approach would have greatly benefited the patient. In addition, I describe a personal case that demonstrates the importance of thought and judgment.

A seventy-year-old woman had an exploratory laparotomy, an operation that peers into the belly to determine the cause of her severe right lower quadrant pain and distension. A perforation of her cecum, the uppermost part of her large intestine, was found, surrounded by a blackened wall of the bowel. A segment of intestine was removed and the pieces of the bowel were reconnected. But the surgeon was so consumed by the need to rid the patient of the leaking intestine that he failed to stop and consider the cause of the leak. The patient remained extremely ill after her procedure. It turned out that a cancer further downstream from the hole had totally obstructed the colon and caused sufficient back pressure to literally blow a hole in the cecum. And so this extremely ill patient required a second operation just a few days later to remove this cancer. Her profoundly complicated postoperative course necessitated a stay of thirty days in the hospital. What, if anything, was the surgeon thinking during the first operation?

In another case, a twenty-five-year-old female medical student came to the emergency room with right lower abdominal pain, fever, and tenderness. A diagnosis of pelvic inflammatory disease was made, because of her pain on examination and because the radiologist believed the CT scan did not show appendicitis. For that reason, an appendectomy was not performed until several days later, when a severe abdominal infection made the diagnosis of appendicitis more obvious. Thankfully, the patient recovered after a very long course, complicated because of the delay in the diagnosis and treatment. Good physicians and surgeons would have considered a wide variety of diseases when confronted with a story such as hers. And life-threatening diagnoses need to be high on the list of possible causes of clinical scenarios. As is often the case, an x-ray report was inappropriately given more importance than a careful history and physical examination.

Thirty years ago, a nineteen-year-old woman came in with massive bright-red rectal bleeding, enough to cause profound shock. A surgeon was consulted, and he removed a one-foot segment of her small intestine. Two months later she had more bleeding, and that prompted a second intestinal resection. The family feared a repetition of the same problem, so I was asked to see the patient. Like a detective, I reviewed the evidence from her two illnesses and operations. It turned out that in both operations, the surgeon had noticed engorged veins draining the intestine. He even dictated a description of this observation in her operative report. With this potential clue to the diagnosis, a pathologist and I looked under the microscope at the tissue removed during the two procedures. The blood vessels were indeed dilated. This fact suggested to me that the large vessels were probably the result of an obstruction to flow. I ordered an angiogram, which confirmed my suspicions.

In order to reduce the pressure in these veins, I performed a shunting operation, diverting some blood away from the intestine. The first surgeon had attributed the bleeding to an inflammatory bowel disease such as Crohn's disease, even though microscopically, it did not have the typical appearance. Furthermore, inflammatory bowel disease rarely causes massive bleeding from the small intestine as seen in this patient. Had a correct diagnosis not been made, tragedy could have ensued. Not long ago, some thirty years after I first cared for this patient, a physician seeing her for a different problem reminded me that she was still free of any hint of intestinal bleeding or difficulties. Knowing of this outcome is a great source of satisfaction to me, and it reminds me again that the surgeon must always be thinking, especially during an operation.

In recent years, more and more value has been given to the results of blood tests and x-rays in place of the surgeon's spending an adequate amount of time or thought in weighing the overall clinical picture. Many of the tests and x-rays are often ordered inappropriately and thus can mislead the physician. Hope springs eternal that one test or another will provide the answer to a diagnostic dilemma, so tests beget tests.

Good surgeons, of course, must be technically adept. However, that is not enough; great technicians who are poor diagnosticians can be dangerous surgeons. An excellent surgeon is one who takes the time to go into depth regarding the symptoms and physical findings in the patient, and who puts together all the facts. Should there be unusual circumstances, then the surgeon must pause to think, "What's wrong with this picture?" It is just as important for a surgeon to know when *not* to operate as when to do so.

Editor's Note: Dr. Silen was my Chief when I was an intern and junior resident in surgery at Harvard Medical School's Beth Israel Hospital. His words of wisdom resonate with me today, as they did when I was a sleepless resident. As I have progressed through my career, I have recognized that the really great surgeons are excellent diagnosticians, not just technicians.

A Life Lived for Others

Mark B. Anderson, MD, FACS

Only a life lived for others is a life worth living.

Albert Einstein

I ALWAYS WANTED to be a doctor. I am not quite sure why. Perhaps it was because my mother always told me that was what I was going to be. Perhaps it was watching numerous episodes of *Medical Center* on television. Either way, it was the right decision. The journey has been filled with many experiences that have shaped my life, both personally and professionally. I expect this fulfillment to continue until the day I retire.

Medical education and training, while comprehensive in most aspects, fails to prepare most physicians for the deeply emotional side of medicine. My training has led me, in part, into the field of cardiopulmonary (heart) transplantation. Transplantation is notorious for being rife with touching stories, and I have many. But after I had been a cardiac surgeon for nine years, having completed medical school and eight years of residency at Lenox Hill Hospital in New York and fellowships in California and Cambridge, England, one story in particular left an indelible mark on my life.

It was the start of the holiday season, and I was on my way to a Christmas party with my daughter. I received an urgent call that one of my colleagues had just been admitted to a nearby hospital with an acute myocardial infarction, or a heart attack. David, another surgeon at the Robert Wood Johnson Medical School in New Jersey, where I was the chief of cardiac surgery, was not doing well. Alone in his house, he had felt chest pain and had the wits to call 911. By the time the ambulance arrived, he was unconscious and near death. My first thought was that there had to be some mistake. He was about my age, young and healthy. And he was a physician, after all. I called back to make sure we were talking about the same person. I was told he was too sick to move to our hospital. I decided to visit David at the hospital that afternoon.

It was soon clear to me that he was in dire straits, and I knew that he would not survive unless he was moved to a hospital where heart surgery was available. He was too sick to *not* be moved. By evening he was in my hospital, the same hospital where David had been a respected physician for fifteen years—the same institution where he had spent countless hours building a surgical program of his own, where he was the chief of the kidney and pancreas transplant surgery program—and he was fighting for his life.

I spent the night with David. His heart just wasn't strong enough to keep pumping blood through his body. The heart attack had weakened it so much that I worried he would not survive the night. By 3 A.M. I decided I had to take him to the operating room to place a ventricular assist device. This relatively new device was needed to support his heart and stabilize his circulation. As a cardiac surgeon, I had done this procedure hundreds of times. Yet I was apprehensive. Normally I would proceed with a respectful fearlessness, a trade necessity. But this time there seemed to be just fear.

I distinctly remember standing at the scrub sink, peering into the room, praying for the ability to focus, to view this as any other case, to not think about how there had been other patients, just as sick, who had not survived this operation or its aftermath. Fortunately, with the help of a great team, the operation went smoothly. The sense of relief for everyone was palpable. Unfortunately, the toughest times were yet to come.

Over the following days, David got worse. His breathing was supported by a ventilator and his kidneys required dialysis. The left ventricular assist device was taking over the work of his heart. Basically, three organs—the lungs, heart, and kidneys—were faltering. Each day numerous visitors would come by his room. Hospital administrators, nurses, colleagues, friends, and family. The entire spectrum of emotions was on display. When a physician becomes the patient, a crippling paralysis seems to take over. Each decision is scrutinized. Everyone has a suggestion. Navigating the minefield of personal emotions and medical decision making is treacherous. A misstep could result in the loss of a friend and colleague, as well as an important fixture in the institution. And my career could be tainted forever. I had to make numerous difficult decisions during this period. It was one of the hardest times in my professional life. What unfolded for me was a transformation of how I viewed myself and how I practiced medicine.

Cardiac surgery is notorious for having many opinionated, stubborn, and seemingly arrogant individuals among its ranks. After all, we cardiac surgeons hold hearts in our hands, and we live with life and death every day. Arrogance is a tradition handed down over generations—one of the "privileges" of being a heart surgeon. To a certain degree, I shared this arrogance. But treating David challenged the mind-set. He was no longer just my patient: he was the collective medical staff's patient. There was no longer any room for individualism. As the reality of this seeped into me, I began to feel a sense of calm, as though a weight had been lifted off my shoulders. It became clear to me that the individuals whom I had most respected in my professional life had been the ones who most respected those around them. I realized that the most effective physicians, and leaders, surrounded themselves with as many talented people as possible. It was time for me to follow the same path.

Unfortunately, despite our best group efforts, David remained critically ill, and it soon became apparent that he would require a heart transplant. David would not survive without a new heart.

As a result, I had to exchange the heart-assisting pump, which was keeping him alive, for another system that could sustain him until a heart was available for transplant—potentially a long time. This second major operation would be especially taxing, given his condition. As we prepared him for surgery, I received a call from the organ procurement organization: a donor had been identified. A heart was available! A million things rushed through my mind. Could he tolerate it? Would there be another donor if we waited?

David was never informed that he would be undergoing a transplant on that day. He didn't even know he was going to wake up with a new heart. After a careful discussion with the entire medical team, we decided to proceed. I went to evaluate and recover (surgically remove) the heart from the donor. Any mistake in this critical procedure could mean the new heart would not work properly when replaced. It was satisfactory—which meant the heart was right for David—and I returned to transplant, or reimplant, the new heart, the most important operation of my career.

Heart transplantation is filled with many conflicts and unknowns. First, there are issues with the donor and the donor family. The donor is surrounded by the terrible grief associated with the loss of a loved one. The loss is nearly always acute and premature. Then there is the difficult decision to donate one's organs. There's the conflict felt by the patient who is facing the end of life. There are issues with the body's accepting the organ—quite literally, a piece of another person. And then recipients—they worry about life after the transplant. Drugs and biopsies to check the health of the new organ will be part of the new life. And behind every day, really every minute, is the possibility of rejection: the cold, hard fact that the new heart, pumping life throughout the body, will be attacked by the body. Viewed as foreign, this new heart is an intruder whose existence is allowed only by the grace of immunosuppressant drugs. And those drugs? These life-giving drugs also cripple the immune system, so that infection or even cancers loom ominously.

Then there are the struggles of the medical team. The surgeon's anxiety over whether the new heart will work, and the real possibility that the surgery will actually make the patient worse. I have experienced all of this—these are the daily tortures haunting a cardiac transplant surgeon. And on this particular day, my struggles were intensified. On that operating table was a friend, a colleague, a surgeon who was needed by thousands of his own patients. On this day, what would the outcome be?

Fortunately, on this day, it would be that all was right. The heart transplant went flawlessly. The diseased heart was removed and sent to pathology, and was replaced with a brand-new, perfectly working specimen.

The ensuing days were filled with a new sense of hope. As David emerged from the haze of his critical illness and surgery, we needed to tell him that he had a new heart. Someone else's heart. I had to tell a transplant surgeon that he was now a *transplant recipient*. Whether David was feeling anger, denial, or disbelief, his initial response was one of disconnection. He seemed not to be able to comprehend the whole sequence of events. That was not surprising though, given the situation. Only as family, friends, and colleagues continued to gather and visit did the pall of what had happened begin to lift. In a similar manner the shroud that had been cast over me began to fall away. I realized that I had been transferring to David all that had been happening to me. The similarities between our lives were too striking for it to have been otherwise. We both had to recover and to rebuild.

Soon David's transformation began, and the subsequent road to recovery was amazing. It was as if he used all his medical experience to heal himself and those around him. I found myself staring at the events and feeling the need to start over as well. Many of those involved needed a new beginning too. And here it was for all of us. He led the way, as he always had in his professional life: with a purpose.

When David felt ready to operate again, he asked me to help him prepare. I went to the operating room and borrowed some instruments. He spent hours practicing—relearning techniques, and refining skills that were embedded in his brain like bicycle riding. It was then that

I understood why I had chosen this field: not because my mother had told me to do so or because I had watched doctor shows on TV. Because practicing medicine was our gift, never to be lost, no matter what happened.

After only three months in recovery and rehabilitation, David returned to practice in triumph. For him, this was the proverbial chance to start over. He could now truly connect with his patients. *He was one of them*, the transplanter becoming the transplantee. He told me a story once of a frightened preoperative kidney transplant patient, concerned about the challenges of his postoperative life. Then David quietly reached into his pocket and pulled out his medication sorter and placed it on the table. David told the patient *his* story. He explained how he was back working, operating, transplanting, more alive than ever. He and the patient formed an immediate connection: its value was immeasurable.

For myself, I felt as though I was now able to leave the ingrained individualism of a heart surgeon behind. I had a fresh view of what it meant to be part of a team, and what it took to be a leader. I had a new sense of confidence in medicine, a new sense of confidence in myself. Gone from my mind were the more traditional teachings and beliefs of generations of surgeons, replaced by a new and exciting outlook on the future of healthcare and my role in it. It was my chance to start over too. I knew the experience would forever change the way I practiced medicine.

With the exception of a heartfelt thank-you, David and I rarely spoke of the events that had transpired. It didn't matter: we each knew how the episode had impacted our lives. I had always felt that he deserved the new heart, the new chance. After all, he had spent his entire professional life committed to the same cause. Yet he would disagree; he expected nothing in return. Nor did I. After all, only a life lived for others is a life worth living.

Editor's Note: Dr. Anderson, the Chief of Cardiac Surgery at my hospital, is one of those doctors that you want to know … just in case you ever need him. Reading this story makes me want to buy him dinner.

In the Service of Two Masters

Lt. Col. Christopher P. Coppola, MD, FACS, Medical Corps, U.S. Air Force

I T IS A sad fact of life that war is an excellent teacher of surgeons. After serving in Iraq and caring for an astounding variety of wounds, I feel well equipped to treat trauma victims. It is true also that the science of surgery advances in bloody lurches when passing through the crucible of war.

Upon graduating from medical school, new doctors take the Hippocratic oath. In 1990, I accepted my commission as an officer in the U.S. military and took an additional oath, as my future wife pinned on my first set of

"butter bars," second lieutenants with the one yellow rect-
angle on each shoulder marking our low rank.

> I, Christopher Coppola, having been appointed
> an officer in the Army of the United States, as
> indicated above in the grade of second lieutenant,
> do solemnly swear that I will support and defend
> the Constitution of the United States against all
> enemies, foreign or domestic, that I will bear true
> faith and allegiance to the same; that I take this
> obligation freely, without any mental reservations
> or purpose of evasion; and that I will well and
> faithfully discharge the duties of the office upon
> which I am about to enter; so help me God.

Since then I have become a pediatric surgeon in
active clinical practice in Texas; I am also a lieutenant
colonel in the Medical Service Corps of the United States
Air Force. As a military surgeon, I am a dual professional.
I am a physician with all the duties and ideals handed
down through traditions that have transcended history
and many cultures. As a United States military officer I
have the added professional responsibility of fulfilling my
duty and remaining true to my oath to defend the Con-
stitution. These weighty responsibilities run deep through
my day-to-day life, and at times can even come into conflict. It is a life in the service of two masters.

My life is a very typical story that could be set in any
of thousands of hometowns across the nation. I am third-

generation Italian American, raised on the shoreline of Connecticut a few miles from where my grandparents first settled in New Haven. My father's successful obstetrics and gynecology practice gave us a life of stability and comfort.

Through witnessing my father's beneficial effect on his patients' lives and the nurturing care my mother gave to our family of four brothers and a sister, I gravitated at an early age to the idea of helping others as a doctor. Since I was the oldest child, I often cared for my siblings and considered becoming a pediatrician, but when I discovered that our Surgeon General C. Everett Koop was a surgeon specifically for children, I knew that I had found my future. I was in high school at the time, and even I realized that all the people who told me that I would probably change my goals along the way had a valid point. Still, twenty-five years later, I have stayed true to that calling. That's longer than I've known my wife.

As college ended, I needed a way to pay for medical school. My parents had generously given me college debt-free, but there were four children after me and it was time I started paying my own bills. I discovered the military's Health Professions Scholarship Program. When I ran the numbers with 1990 tuition fees and surgeons' salaries, I realized that financially I could pay off school loans a lot quicker than I could complete a military obligation, but by that point I had become interested in military service for nonfinancial reasons. Like many other youths I had been inspired by President Ronald Reagan to patriotism and an awareness of the great advantages we are given as U.S.

citizens. During college I studied in Spain, and it amazed me that a country that had high levels of unemployment and fewer governmental services than the United States required a year of military service from all young people. I developed a conviction that it was only right that I give something back to my country in thanks for the great fortune of calling the USA my home. I signed on with the United States Air Force.

My time commitment to the military during medical school was minor. Each year I would complete a month-long rotation on one of the Air Force bases that had a hospital. My first rotation was the Health Professions Officer Indoctrination Course. This was a highly softened version of basic training given to young doctors in training. We were second lieutenants. The enlisted troops in officer-candidate school, with whom we shared Medina Training Annex in San Antonio, Texas, would chuckle at our uniform faux pas. They would spread out just enough as they walked by us that we had to awkwardly return a salute to every single one of them in turn. Their course of training was much harder, but even then in the combined enlisted/officer's club these same men who poked fun at us would confide that crooked uniform or not, one of the most important confidence builders to a war fighter is the presence of skillful physicians ready to care for any battle wounds.

One of our lecturers was a general who had been decorated as both a surgeon and a pilot in the Vietnam War. When asked how he justified the conflict between being a healer and serving in combat, he responded,

"Some people need curing; some people need killing."
He asserted that the role of officer must come before
duties of a physician in wartime. This statement troubled
me deeply, and even though it was early in my career, I
knew in my heart that I would always be a physician first
and an officer second.

During my first year of medical school at Johns Hopkins, President George H. W. Bush sent troops to the Middle East in Operation Desert Storm. My classmate Dave,
who was also on military scholarship, and I watched the
brief war unfold on television, wondering if we would be
pulled for duty. When I reported in to my command, they
made it clear that a half-trained doctor wouldn't be much
use to them and I should just keep up with my studies.

Surgical training is long, and pediatric surgical training is even longer. I started residency in 1994 and finished
my pediatric surgery fellowship in 2003. Part of my training was at the Veterans Administration (VA) Hospital in
West Haven, Connecticut. It was a joy to care for the
aging World War II veterans and hear stirring stories of
war and love from these members of "the Greatest Generation." Although the conditions and inefficiency at the VA
could be frustrating, I always felt honored helping those
who had given so much to keep our country great. I had
originally committed to four years of military service in
exchange for a medical school scholarship, but I had to
commit an additional two years to be permitted to train
as a pediatric surgeon. I had been a military officer since
1990 yet had never been assigned to a military base. It was

a foregone conclusion that I would be assigned to Wilford Hall in Texas, since it is the only Air Force hospital that provides pediatric surgery. In 2003 I my wife and I moved our family of five to San Antonio to begin a new life.

It was my responsibility to provide all the pediatric surgical needs for the military families who came to Wilford Hall for their medical care. This population wasn't just limited to San Antonio; I treated patients whose parents were stationed at military bases across Texas, Louisiana, and Oklahoma. At times I even received children who had been medically evacuated from Central America, Europe, and even as far away as Japan. I learned that part of the promise the military makes to the troops is that their families will get medical care, no matter how far-flung their global assignments. Military families never failed to impress me with their grace and discipline. Without complaint they would drive three hours from Fort Hood in Killeen, Texas, just to have me check their child's incision and remove stitches. It is a privilege to treat any family, but I felt a special honor acting as physician to those who had pledged to make the sacrifices that are necessary when one serves in the military.

As a military surgeon I had the chance to complete medical missions that I never would have seen in the civilian world. Our hospital had the only worldwide deployable extracorporeal membrane oxygenation (ECMO) circuit and team. ECMO is a technical term for artificial lung and heart support, similar to the bypass used by cardiothoracic surgeons performing open heart surgery. We use this technique on newborns with severe pulmonary ailments such as congenital diaphragmatic hernia and pulmonary hypertension. Our team could fly anywhere in the world on military aircraft, attach a dying child to the ECMO circuit, and then bring the child home to San Antonio for definitive treatment. As the surgeon on the team, I found it an odd experience to fly ten hours to Hawaii, perform a twenty-minute operation to insert a tiny tube into the blood vessels in a baby's neck, and then fly another ten hours home. I would boast that I was the laziest member of the team, working for twenty minutes and taking up space for twenty hours. The patients were often amazed that we would commit a mission of fifteen people and an expenditure of hundreds of thousands of dollars to rescue their child. We were proud to be able to provide this specialized care to service members' children no matter how far from home the military sent them.

I have twice deployed to Iraq in support of Operation Iraqi Freedom. While I was deployed, I staffed the Air Force Theater Hospital in Balad, Iraq. When I deploy, my tasking is not as a pediatric surgeon but as a combat support trauma surgeon ready to treat wounds sustained in battle. At our hospital in Iraq we treated Coalition troops, Iraqi security forces, contractors, enemy combatants, and civilians, including children. It was a shocking experience to see firsthand the devastating fragmentation injuries and high-velocity projectile wounds that are the hallmark of modern combat. Often the Black Hawk helicopters transporting patients from the site of a blast would deliver soldiers, detainees, and civilians on the same trip. At our hospital, all comers received the same level of care: the best we could give. There were times when we received so many patients that we operated on six patients at once in our three operating rooms continuously for periods of thirty-six hours or more. With the unpredictable nature of war, these periods of intense activity would alternate with times when we would loiter around the hospital with nothing to do but exercise or read email from home. As part of our staff of three hundred, including many surgical subspecialists, I felt like I was part of an enthusiastic, cooperative team. I knew I could count on my brothers and sisters in arms no matter what challenge came down the pike.

My colleagues and I were able to publish several observations accrued at the combat support hospital, building on the achievements of military surgeons before us, stretching back to the Revolutionary War in the United States and much further back around the globe.

I have also had the great privilege to provide some humanitarian pediatric surgical care to Iraqi children with nontraumatic conditions. Once word got out to the local population that there was a pediatric surgeon at the base, parents began bringing children to the gate asking if they could be treated at the hospital.

During my deployments, I did not like being away from the family I love so dearly. My burden of two short deployments, however, was much easier than the long multiple tours to the Middle East that so many troops are completing. I found the busy times sad because of the crippling and lethal injuries we saw, and the idle times difficult because of the longing to be home. But I always felt useful, needed, and certain that the services I provided were deeply appreciated. I do not regret having served my country in wartime, but there are memories I would give up if I could. We call time at the hospital in Iraq "the million-dollar experience you wouldn't pay a dime for."

Back on U.S. soil, I make myself useful again caring for the children of service members. Our base is responsible for the basic military training of young men and women entering active duty, so each Friday I see a fresh crop of the newest airmen in the Air Force graduating from their training. Soon my commitment to the military will be up and I will transition to civilian practice. There is nothing that could convince me to continue my tenure in the military, but I know that there are aspects of my service that I will miss for a long time to come.

The time will come for me to give up my profession as officer and give full allegiance to my deeper calling as a physician. I feel a fuller love and appreciation for my country now that I have served and probably too because I have grown older. I am proud that I had the opportunity to serve, and I know that I could serve a hundred years and still not repay the great gift that has been given to us by citizens and patriots before us. We are all fortunate that there are young men and women who are willing to step up and give service in the military as those like me step down, because that is our greatest resource and will keep our country strong and free.

Editor's Note: The story of surgeons in the military is one that is not heard often. It is an unfortunate fact that war advances the field of surgery rapidly, by necessity. Dr. Coppola's service to the country is greatly appreciated.

Intangible Rewards

Robert T. Grant, MD, FACS

IT ISN'T OFTEN that a plastic surgeon can point to a specific patient and say, "I saved that man's life!" I'm not talking about taking out someone's appendix or fixing a patient's coronary arteries after a heart attack. I took action (outside of the operating room) that literally made the difference in one man's survival.

John had undergone open heart surgery and developed a sternal wound infection. This complication is one of the most feared after heart surgery, and John's cardiac disease had already made him chronically ill. As a diabetic, he was sick and frail, just the type of person at risk for a serious infection. After I routed out his infected, rotting breastbone and ribs and reconstructed his infected chest wall, his health began to recover. Then one day about a month after leaving the hospital, he returned to my office with a fluid collection under the skin of his chest. When I drained the fluid, I noted that it was bloodier than it should have been, but this was not too uncommon. A few days later, the fluid had reaccumulated and I drained it again. His blood pressure and pulse rate were in the normal range and his blood counts were not too much changed from where they had been in the past. But something just did not look right to me. He also expressed his sense of "impending doom" to me, saying he just felt "something" was wrong. I called his cardiologist and heart surgeon. Both had seen John recently and reassured me he was fine. But he didn't pass my own personal "look test."

Normally, I would have arranged for some outpatient testing, perhaps a CT scan of the operated area. But for some reason I decided to admit John to the hospital directly from my office. I wanted to get him in the hospital fast to expedite the scheduling and completion of the diagnostic workup I had in mind. Ten minutes after he arrived on the hospital ward, I got a call from his admitting nurse. "Your patient's blood pressure is ninety and he looks awful," she said. I rushed right over from my office. As I began to evaluate John I noted how bad he looked—pale, almost lifeless. The fluid that I had just removed was again present under the skin of his chest. And before my eyes, he suddenly went into cardiac arrest. I immediately began CPR and a cardiac code was called. He wasn't responding and the fluid under his skin was expanding, making the chest-compressions part of CPR difficult to administer. I told the nurse to get someone from cardiac surgery. I then made the difficult decision to open John's chest.

Open cardiac massage—physically using one's hand to squeeze the blood from the heart, like a cook emptying water out of a kitchen sponge—is a particularly effective kind of CPR. But usually it can be done only when the patient is in the open-heart operating room or perhaps in the emergency room right after the patient sustains a knife or gunshot wound that rips into the heart. Doing what I was doing was very unusual for any doctor other than a cardiothoracic surgeon. But it had to be done. This was life or death.

When I got into his chest cavity, I immediately saw the problem. John's weakened, thinned, scarred heart muscle had ruptured in an area where he had suffered a previous heart attack, leaving a hole through which his body's blood supply was leaking. The fluid I had drained earlier was actual blood and fluid that sometimes surrounds the heart after surgery. I realized that he had been suffering from a *sentinel bleed*; like a leak in a dam before the dam collapses, this was the little bleed that presaged the full disaster. I grabbed a clamp and was able to close the hole temporarily. I continued to compress his heart—squeezing out that blood and giving the heart a few seconds to refill, then squeezing again while the team poured fluids and blood into John's veins as fast as was physically possible. I was his human assisted heart pump, and I hoped I was pumping enough to keep his brain and other organs alive.

The cardiac surgery team arrived in short order (after all, they wanted to know who had the nerve to open a man's chest) and took over from there. They did a masterful job in repairing the ruptured cardiac aneurysm and managing the complex medical problems, which took weeks to resolve.

Happily, John recovered completely, his mind and body scarred but mended following his near-death experience. As he is better, John doesn't have to stop by the hospital as much anymore. In one of his postop visits, he asked me what made me keep him around and not send him home. We both know he surely would have collapsed and died had he gone home. I told him, "I guess it was just my years of training, experience, and instinct." But I know I got lucky too. And even years later, it's no secret that I always enjoy when he stops by my office to say hello and thank you!

Another patient, Dan, made an appointment to see me recently. When I got into the exam room I noticed in the paperwork that he had listed me as his surgeon from two decades earlier. It was right after I had started my own clinical practice. I remembered little of his case, even though it had to be one of the first I had managed as an "attending surgeon"—the real deal after completion of my residency and fellowship training. I had performed microvascular surgery—techniques that use microscopic stitches and tiny instruments under a microscope to move tissue from one area of the body to another. Thirty-five years ago he would have required an amputation, but with the tools of a plastic surgeon I had moved a piece of muscle down to Dan's heel, covering up a bone fracture that had become infected after it was repaired orthopedically. These kinds of fractures are notoriously difficult to heal. Even if the infection is controlled, sometimes arthritis and chronic inflammation set in, often leaving the injured person with a lifelong hobble or even a wheelchair existence.

While I had little recall of the circumstances surrounding the procedure and his excellent and total recovery, Dan certainly had no problems recalling every event that had transpired after his accident and during his recovery. He reminded me of details of my professional life and interactions I had long forgotten. He spoke of my relationships, where I was going on work and personal travel, and how much he believed in me and what I was doing for him. It was a fun trip down memory lane for me. In fact, he had come in not for any real medical reason but just to thank me. You see, he was *walking* his daughter down the aisle that next Saturday. He just wanted me to know how grateful he was that, thanks to me, it was going to happen just like he and his daughter had always wanted.

Every winter I wear a very characteristic scarf. It's handwoven, with some bright wool colors and a great texture. It feels wonderful against my neck and does a fantastic job keeping out the cold. It was a gift from another patient on whom I performed sophisticated reconstructive leg surgery, with a superb outcome. Every time I am complimented on how good I look wearing the scarf, I relive the deeply personal thanks and appreciation of this patient. The heartfelt rewards and handmade gifts from patients are so much more valuable than any appraisal of their intrinsic worth!

It's called the *practice* of surgery because a surgeon is always learning and improving his skills. I have grown and progressed during my years in practice. Growth comes from knowledge and experience. Surgeons improve technically and develop better judgment not only from the hours, weeks, months, and years of patient care, but also from exposure to things not part of one's background.

The popular media today portray plastic surgeons in a less than flattering light, as seemingly preoccupied more with their own egos and financial interests than with the concerns of their patients. My life as a practicing plastic surgeon is much more rewarding, rich, and enjoyable than that of the characters portrayed on TV or in the movies. I've been a plastic surgeon for over twenty-five years, and the personal and professional satisfaction from caring for patients continues to inspire me every day.

Editor's Note: I first met Dr. Grant when we were medical students in Albany in 1978, and we reconnected again as residents at Cornell. Nearly three decades later, Bob is the Chief at Cornell and Columbia, and we're still working together.

A Fat Boy's Dream

George A. Fielding, MD, FRCS, FRACS

IDECIDED TO BE a surgeon like my dad when I was ten years old. I just liked the way he smelled when he came home—antiseptic, ether, and chloroform—and the way he looked in his white coat. I also liked the fact that he made sick people better. I used to drive around with him on weekends while he went from hospital to hospital doing his rounds, and he'd chat to me about football and movies and history, but occasionally about patients. Sometimes I'd see him cry, when a long-term patient died from her breast cancer. I liked the boxes of fruit we got at Christmas from grateful patients. I fell in love with my nurse when I had my appendix out when I was twelve, and I thought it'd be cool to work with beautiful, kind women.

As I grew older, I worked hard, got into medical school in Brisbane, Australia, did a surgical residency, and became a surgeon in 1986.

In 1989 I'd been working in England for two years doing fellowships first in pancreatic surgery and then in colorectal surgery. One otherwise unimportant day, a friend told me about a surgeon in Lyons, France, who was taking gallbladders out via a laparoscope. Through a tube! Through a tube with a lens at the end of it that the surgeon could use to look into the belly without making a long incision. My mother-in-law, a tiny woman, had recently had her gallbladder removed through a hole so big I could put my head in. It took her six months to get over it. I figured this new method might be a better way. I'd moved to Bern, Switzerland, to do a six-month liver surgery fellowship with the great Dr. Les Blumgart when I caught the train to visit Dr. Philippe Mouret in Lyons. Dr. Mouret was the first to use this technique, and it changed surgery forever. I was the first Anglo to visit him, was amazed by what I saw, and there and then decided that this was the way forward. And it was. Since 1990 I've done more than 15,000 laparoscopic operations, and I love what I do to this day.

Most of all, I love doing surgery to treat obesity. I'd like to tell you why I do laparoscopic surgery for obesity, why it matters so much.

Everybody dreams. What do obese people dream about? Sex, of course, everyday fears, weird things, just like everyone else. Above all else, though, they dream about being thin, not being hungry, and looking normal. Many millions of obese people have this dream but only a few have it come true. Even fewer have it stay true.

Why is it so hard to lose weight? The problem boils down to two forces—mathematics and hunger.

Take the easy one first, mathematics. Eat more than you burn, and you'll gain weight. Simple, but devastating.

Hunger is trickier. The hypothalamus is deep in the brain's most primitive part, and deeper still is the satiety center. When it doesn't work correctly, the center always sends the same message: that we have not had enough to eat. We never feel full; we are always hungry. *This* is the root of obesity. Thin people, who are typically born to be thin and stay thin, respond appropriately to the stimulus of being full by stopping eating. That's how they stay thin. On the other hand, obese people spend their lives trying to control hunger. They diet, they starve, and they face obstacles to their willpower every day, all the time surrounded by food. In the 1980s a study revealed that fat people would rather lose a leg or an eye than be fat, and they would rather be a thin pauper than a fat millionaire. Why? Because they know what everybody thinks. Would America elect a fat president?

In 1991 the U.S. National Institutes of Health (NIH) reviewed 4,500 publications on weight loss and found that the maximum sustainable weight loss by *any* diet, exercise, or behavioral modification program is twenty-five pounds. That's two dress sizes! You can keep twenty pounds off, but you will virtually never, ever, ever keep fifty, a hundred, or two hundred pounds off because the hunger will always get you. So, what to do? Well, either you keep trying and go mad; give up, get fatter, and go mad; or have an operation.

The second major finding of the NIH was that surgery is the only treatment for morbid obesity that works. And so surgery is now encouraged. By NIH guidelines, 10 percent of the population of Australia, the United States, the United Kingdom, and Europe are eligible for obesity surgery. Now try picturing such a large number of people. Ten percent of the adult population of the USA is the population of New York City, or the entire population of Australia! The only known cure—yes, cure—for diabetes, sleep apnea, and asthma is weight loss. The only known, proven long-term path to weight loss greater than twenty-five pounds is surgery. A lot of people need this surgery.

Obese people have surgery for one reason—to be not obese anymore. The driving force behind the decision varies. Wanting a healthy life, avoiding multiple medications, fear of early death. Wanting to be alive for their families, play with their children, get a job, get a promotion, get pregnant, have a child, sleep without a CPAP sleep apnea mask. Wanting to have their spouse able to sleep in the same room because the snoring has stopped! Normal life. Like fitting in a movie seat, a plane seat, a toilet seat, or a bus seat. Not to mention walking up five stairs, up the street, out of the house, anywhere without gasping, or going to the beach, the gym, or a dress shop without feeling like a freak show.

How do I know all this? Easy. In the last twelve years I have operated on over five thousand morbidly obese patients in Brisbane and New York and I've heard it all five thousand times. They just want a life. Sure they're scared, sure it's a big step, but hell, nothing else has worked. So they come in, nervous, a deep part of them sure it's a con like everything else, ready for failure yet desperate for success. Eventually I tell them okay, I'll do it. Often they just cry. Why on earth would they cry? Relief that it is actually going to happen, that someone believes they have tried, that they don't have to do another stupid, doomed diet. So they cry.

How else do I know? Also easy—I'm one of them. I've had the surgery too. It's weird hearing five thousand people tell you your own life story.

I was the fat kid in grade school. I saw my first doctor to see if I had an endocrine gland problem when I was ten. I didn't. I just ate too much, so I was put on my first diet. It was torture. I cheated all the time, because I was starving. I was very active, played all the sports, and was also quite brainy. We never had TV, so I read a lot and played music. I just ate all the time. Clothes were a problem. Nothing fit, so Mum made them specially for me. I was called every imaginable simile and metaphor for fat. Not surprisingly, I became completely determined to beat all the bastards. I lived starving hungry.

I have a beautiful wife and four great kids. I became a surgeon by age twenty-nine and was in private practice by age thirty-four. I played rugby quite well and later coached, and played two musical instruments well enough to be in a band until I was forty-three. I read thousands of books, listened to endless music, traveled the world, surfed at Australia's Noosa from the time I was twelve, bought a share in a house in Burgundy, France, and drank more great wine than was strictly necessary. I simply took life by the throat. I find surgery a joy. I've operated as a guest surgeon in Britain, France, Japan, Singapore, Hong Kong, Bangkok, and the USA. I love teaching, am not backward in coming forward, surely appear arrogant to many, and make laparoscopic surgery look as hard as pulling on socks.

But despite my drive and all these accomplishments, I just could not stop eating. I could never control my hunger. The pain and humiliation of always being hungry, and always fighting it, just exhausted me. Despite living a life where false modesty has been a wasted emotion, deep down I felt a failure.

Since 1980 I have lost more than seventy pounds, four times. Each time took about eighteen months. I felt like a different person each time: strong, confident, aggressive, in control. Then—whoosh—blink and it's all back on, plus some. Try being two hundred pounds, then being three hundred pounds. You still think like the two-hundred-pound tough guy, but you look and feel like a big, smart, aggressive blimp. Imagine Big Pussy, not Tony Soprano. So you start back on the road, dieting, running, working too hard, overcompensating in everything to override how awful you feel.

This was the cycle of my life for twenty years.

Then I got sick—all kinds of sick. Asthma, reflux, hypertension, high cholesterol, sleep apnea, depression, and finally atrial fibrillation and ventricular heart arrhythmias. I was forty-two years old, on ten tablets a day, in the middle of a midlife crisis to end them all, and I thought I was going to die. I was working like a lunatic, out of breath all the time, tired all the time, going a bit crazy.

In addition to performing my usual surgeries, I was also doing ten bariatric (weight loss) operations a week, putting in little silicone devices called Lap-Bands that restrict the amount of food that can go into the stomach; and doing gastric bypasses, operations that rearrange the plumbing of the gut in a way that would make Rube Goldberg proud. I had been converted to the cause four years previously, and was very happy with the results. This was the most satisfying work I had done in my career—making people healthy and happy, giving them a normal life. The patients' stories were all the same as mine. But I held off on having the surgery myself.

One day I gave in to the pressure, weighed myself, and nearly fainted at the figure: 310 pounds. I sat down and rang my friend Paul O'Brien in Melbourne and booked myself in for a Lap-Band. I took control.

Many doctors have written about being on the "other side," on the receiving end of medical treatment. We all find it an awkward place. As a group, surgeons are famed for their inability to give in, to admit frailty. As an old patient once said, "The only difference between God and a surgeon is that God doesn't think he's a surgeon." Flying to Melbourne to have the surgery, I was scared, nervous about my powerlessness, anxious about complications. But I was thrilled to be gaining control. I'd seen the procedure help so many of my own patients. I would gain control, for certain.

And I have—nine years out, no hunger, and one hundred pounds down. I feel great, am off all my pills, have boundless energy to do anything I want without getting tired. One night in the hospital, three days off work, five tiny cuts in my belly, eating slowly, eating small meals, never being hungry. That's the biggest blessing, *never being hungry*. Hunger no longer rules my world. A fat boy's dream has come true.

Editor's Note: Dr. George Fielding has the world's largest experience in Lap-Band surgery. His Program for Surgical Weight Loss at NYU has become the nation's busiest. In less than a half an hour, his surgery gives people "a shot at a normal life", as he told me.

LIFE WAS GREAT

Lawrence S. Zachary, MD, FACS

I HAD BEEN an attending surgeon and a full-time faculty member at the University of Chicago (also known as "the Harvard of the Midwest") for two and a half years. I was doing everything I had ever dreamed of doing: microsurgery, hand surgery, breast reconstruction, and even some cosmetic surgery. I was teaching medical students and residents and I was part of a research program. Life was great. Until one Monday.

It was January 2, 1989, a holiday because New Year's Day had fallen on Sunday. A young boy had cut his hand at home and I was needed at the hospital to repair his wounds. Coming in to the hospital on a holiday was just part of my duties as a plastic and reconstructive surgeon. I had been doing exactly that for years, even during my plastic surgery residency. All was normal that day as I arrived at the hospital and went through all my usual routines. I introduced myself; looked at the cut; gathered a nurse, instruments, and sutures; and then scrubbed my hands. I fixed the cut on the boy's hand with my usual meticulous surgical technique and then talked to the family. I scribbled the obligatory hospital paperwork, washed my hands, grabbed my coat, got in my car, and headed to the store. Friends were coming over, and my wife had given me a list of things to buy.

Then my life changed forever.

I pulled out of the hospital's parking garage, passed through a quiet intersection under a green light, and then it happened. A car coming from my left went through the red light at about fifty-five miles per hour and struck my car broadside, blasting into my door. With an explosion of light and sound, my car was crushed, upended, and launched into a ditch. It turned out the other driver had dropped his cigarettes on the floor and was picking them up. *His cigarettes!*

The driver of the other car was barely hurt. But me—I had to be extracted from the car with the "jaws of life." I was rushed to a trauma center four miles from the hospital where I had just been working, because my hospital had given up their "Trauma One" status as of January 1—just my luck. The ER doctors, my colleagues, stabilized me. They placed a tube in my chest to reexpand my collapsed lung. As the blood poured out of my head lacerations, the doctor squelched the bleeding by sewing me up. There was the irony: I was the one supposed to be doing the sewing. They placed a breathing tube in my trachea to help bring oxygen to my battered lungs. I had also broken my pelvis, an injury that can be deadly. But that wasn't even the worst of it: I had also sustained closed head trauma, a major brain injury.

I was in a coma. It was not clear to my doctors what my level of function would be *if* I came out of the coma. Many in my situation do not. They just lie around for days, weeks, even months until infection finally chews away at their tissues, claiming another victim. After eight days I emerged from my coma into consciousness. My wife was called; she rushed to the hospital and into my room to find me strapped in a chair, drooling and unable to talk or walk.

I have been asked numerous times since then: Did I see a white light when I was in a coma? I did not. I have no memory of the accident; in fact, I have amnesia from before the event and don't remember anything from the prior week. All the details, everything I just explained about the accident, was told to me by my friends and family. The first three months after the accident are a blur.

Ultimately, I spent three weeks in the intensive care unit and then two months at a rehabilitation hospital. After the accident, I had difficulty speaking clearly, and the right-brain injury affected the motor skills of my left leg, which made walking difficult. Amazingly my intellect, cognitive abilities, and memory were intact; my arms and hands were not affected by the accident, and my fine motor skills were not impaired.

When I was a patient in the hospital, doctors and nurses would ask me what I planned to do after I returned home. I would tell them, "I am going to be a plastic surgeon." They would smile and nod, then walk away. I know they felt pity, thinking I would be playing Bingo and watching television for the rest of my years. I finally left the hospital after twelve long weeks—only to remain an outpatient at a rehabilitation center for another year.

No one believed I would ever return to being a surgeon. My wife was told I would be limited in my ability to function. When she, in turn, told me this, I informed her I *was* going to return to my practice. She understood: she knew I would not feel like a complete person unless I could be a plastic surgeon again. It was my life. It was who I am. It was what I spent over a decade training to do. I *was* a plastic surgeon, and I would be one again.

The dean of the University of Chicago Medical Center said he did not want a brain-injured physician on the hospital staff. The chief of plastic surgery convinced him to let me go through a supervised "retread" program. If I failed, the university and hospital administrators would be able to claim they gave me a chance.

It was a long, arduous process. I spent two more years going through a program of graduated surgical responsibility. I had a committee of outside plastic surgeons, not affiliated with the University of Chicago, evaluate my performance. I even had to take an IQ test. *I* knew I was still

Larry Zachary. *I* knew my intellect was intact, and *I* knew I could still operate and take care of my patients. I just had to convince everyone else.

I passed the outside evaluation with flying colors. So now *everyone,* including the university, finally knew that Larry Zachary was back. Oh, and the IQ test? It showed my IQ had gone *up.*

After three years, three months, and eight days (but who's counting?) of being out of practice on disability, I was reinstated as a plastic and reconstructive surgeon at my "Harvard of the Midwest."

Twenty years have passed since my accident. Life is not the same, but life is good. I function well and am an active surgeon. My speech, however, never returned to normal.

My patients and I now have a special bond. On our first meetings, I tell every patient that my speech was affected by an accident and if they don't understand what I have told them, they should say so and I will repeat it. Some people tell me I have an accent and ask where I am from. I tell them Brussels, because most people have no idea what a person from Brussels sounds like.

I think my patients appreciate that *I* have been a patient and I know what it is like to go through trauma, surgery, and recovery. I've been on the other side. I've been as close to dying as one can be without actually doing so. And I'm now back in action. Am I the same person? Of course, but my life has been forever changed. When asked for advice, I tell people the inspirational slogans "Life is great" and "Never give up." And also to be sure to buy a car with side air bags, and don't forget the disability insurance. Just in case.

Editor's Note: Dr. Larry Zachary's account of his near tragedy and his recovery is inspiring. I trained with Dr. Zachary at the University of Chicago and was one of the many hundreds who silently prayed for him during his ordeal.

The Smile's in the Mail

Yuman Fong, MD, FACS

I WORK IN A tertiary cancer center. Two-thirds of the patients I see for surgery come from a distance of greater than two hundred miles. So it is not surprising that every day of every week I receive multiple packets in the mail containing medical records, CDs with various scans, and letters asking the same question: "Can you help us?" If it seems very impersonal, that's because it is meant to be. Physicians don't want to tell a patient sitting in front of them that nothing can be done—especially if the patient has come thousands of miles.

Early spring is a particularly hard time to receive these mail calls for help. The cheerful time of year, colored by new flowers and clear blue skies, juxtaposes with the dire situation of many patients stricken by cancer. As I opened yet another large envelope on such a spring afternoon, a wallet-sized school picture fell out. The back side was facing up, and it read simply, "This is my little girl, please help her live." When I turned over the picture, a smiling, beautiful twelve-year-old looked back at me. I remember thinking: please let it be a resectable case, treatable with surgery.

Ashley was a "flyer" on her junior high school cheer-leading team. (I didn't know what that was either, at the time.) It turns out the flyer is the cheerleader at the top of the pyramid, who is tossed way up in the air and performs the most acrobatic of maneuvers. So when she had a hard landing one day and complained of pain in her upper abdomen, everyone thought it was just a muscular injury. But the pain didn't improve. Many tests were done, eventually revealing a large liver cancer that had grown into the largest vein of the body, called the vena cava, and the heart. She was declared unresectable—and therefore terminal—and placed on chemotherapy.

Hepatocellular carcinoma is a common cancer that usually arises in the liver of patients with cirrhosis. More than a million cases will occur this year, mainly in Southeast Asia or Africa, where viral hepatitis is common. In America, this cancer is already unusual. Having it occur in an otherwise healthy teenager is even rarer. Cancer is always unfortunate, but cancer in the very young is tragic.

One of the drugs used to treat this cancer is Adriamy-cin™, which poisons the heart. While the chemotherapy managed to control Ashley's cancer for a time, the treatments had taken a toll. Ashley's body was no longer tolerating treatments, and her parents had begun sending out desperate cries for help.

I called her mom, whose handwriting covered the back of the photograph. I told her Ashley's tumor was probably removable—but would require removal of half the liver, part of the vena cava, and part of the heart. I also mentioned the possibility that her daughter might die on the operating table. It is hard to discuss these things on the phone with someone you have never met, but it is even harder to do in front of a twelve-year-old patient. I also bring these difficult issues up in advance because it is very tough for parents to make the right decision if they are confronted with the information only a few days before the scheduled surgery, thousands of miles from home.

"We have done a lot of research," she said in her deliberate midwestern manner. "You come highly recommended. We trust you. Go do the right thing. God will then choose what happens."

Ashley and her parents arrived a few weeks later and stayed at the church next door to the hospital. As they had no other family nearby, the pastor there and the religious community were of great comfort to them in those stressful times. I met Ashley early one Monday morning. She had lost all her hair from the chemotherapy. She looked different from her picture—until she smiled. The treatment had not robbed her of her warmth, her humor, or her spirit. "Let's go," she said in the tone of a cheerleader. "I'm ready."

The surgery went well, technically: four hours; no transfusion needed. Ashley's postoperative recovery was harder. Her life-preserving chemotherapy had given her a seventy-year-old heart; managing her fluids and heart function was as tricky as for a septuagenarian. After some anxious days, though, she was on her way to recovering completely. She was out of the hospital in two weeks and was ready to fly home a week later.

Before she left, Ashley came in for a final checkup and to say goodbye. She and her mom asked the usual questions. What should she eat? What are her restrictions? I had a longer than usual chat with them. I told them that how much her heart recovered was likely to be the most important determinant of restrictions. I was not worried about the liver, since it was likely to already have completely grown back. I did not mention my biggest worry: that the cancer might return. I made her promise to return to cheerleading, and said goodbye.

When patients come from far away, it is not unusual not to hear any further news. It's both good and bad: no news is better than bad news. A year later I did call Ashley's local oncologist, who told me that Ashley was doing quite well. She was off treatments and almost completely back to the life of a teenager. I happily returned to my work that day and did not think of this case again for years.

Then, six years later, it arrived: the envelope with Ashley's return address in the upper left corner. It sat untouched on my desk all afternoon. After I had made all the important clinical decisions of the day, I worked up the courage to reach for the letter. And there it was: a wallet-sized photo of a beautiful woman. She was all grown up but still had the same smile. She had written because she was getting ready to go off to college. The accompanying letter was a page of plans, hopes, and aspirations, just like an eighteen-year-old is supposed to have.

That week, reviewing the cases that arrived by mail was easier than usual. As I read each tragic story, I imagined the beautiful smiles that we may be able to preserve with lifesaving surgery.

Editor's Note: This story exemplifies why Dr. Fong was my best intern when I was at Cornell. He has lived up to all expectations as the "liver guy" at Sloan-Kettering. I appreciated Dr. Fong's skills even more when he operated on a relative of mine two decades later.

Mohammed's Plight

Ronald S. Weiss, MD

MY FIRST ENCOUNTER with Mohammed began mundanely enough when I received a phone call at the office from a colleague I had known for several years, an emergency medicine physician whom I held in particularly high regard. He told me about a basketball buddy of his, a volunteer who was an advocate for refugees for the nonprofit Exodus World Service. Exodus helps churches in the Chicago area aid the displaced from around the globe. He told me about a Somalian who had lived in a refugee camp for fifteen years and was about to be sent back to Africa because he was blind. In order to be admitted into the United States, a refugee has to employable. Because Mohammed was a married father of three daughters, the whole family was in jeopardy of being sent back to Somalia. I immediately agreed to volunteer to see Mohammed, but I certainly was not optimistic about his prognosis. His deadline for being deported was approaching soon, so I agreed to see him immediately.

Mohammed stood tall in my office, accompanied by his basketball-playing advocate from Exodus and an interpreter. In his mid-fifties, Mohammed appeared much older, and I was immediately taken by his quiet dignity. As I examined him, it was obvious that he had no vision—but did have light perception in his right eye and hand motion perception in his left. As I focused on the right eye, I realized that he had severe end-stage glaucoma, with elevated eye pressures and a destroyed optic nerve—and no chance for visual recovery.

His left eye housed a cataract so dense that no light could penetrate to the retina. Surgery on cataracts, while now a simple outpatient procedure performed on millions each year, miraculously restored vision in blind people when first performed in 1748. Although I could not examine the vital functioning parts of the eye, Mohammed's eye pressure was normal and his optic nerve did appear to be functioning; so, with a glimmer of optimism, I agreed to donate my surgical time to perform the complicated cataract surgery. Seeking the support of the hospital to donate their operating facilities and surgical staff would be more difficult.

Fortunately, I had just cured a chronic, complex eye problem in the wife of the hospital's new CEO. She came by the office that week to drop off a small gift, and in the course of our conversation I told her about Mohammed's plight. Within forty-five minutes I received a call from her husband, who offered the hospital facilities. I called Mohammed's advocate at Exodus, gave him the good news, and arranged for a surgical date as I began to ponder the surgical techniques I would use for this intricate case.

Even on the day of the procedure, I had no idea whether Mohammed would have any improvement in his vision after the operation. I prepared the eye and was ready to make my incision. I had removed thousands of cataracts during my residency at the University of Chicago and nearly two decades in practice, but even that gave me no solace—this cataract was the densest, most difficult one I had ever seen. Fortunately, our hospital had the latest technology, and I was able to remove the cataract without difficulty and precisely insert an artificial lens implant. When a patient with vision in only one eye has surgery, I do not patch the seeing eye but only shield it. The shield has pinholes to see through to provide immediate vision. However, Mohammed had not had any vision in either eye for a long time, and I wanted to ensure the utmost safety. Therefore, I decided to patch and shield the eye, adding to the next day's drama.

I always see my patients the morning following surgery. This day, the patient was not alone: he had an entourage consisting of his advocate, his interpreter, his wife, and his three daughters. Along with this troupe came my entire office staff, all of whom wanted to be actively involved in this special case. Mohammed's wife led him in, with the whole crew in tow. I knew that the surgery had gone well, but I honestly did not know if he would have any vision at all. I knew how much was at stake for this family, who had always been so respectful to each other as well as to everyone around them. It was obvious they cared deeply for each other and were themselves extremely nervous for their patriarch.

As I began to slowly remove the shield and patch, I felt butterflies in the pit of my stomach. I had found myself over the past several weeks often discussing Mohammed and the life he had led. I knew that either he was able to see, get a job, and stay in this country, or the whole family was going back to their brutal life in Africa. The patch and shield were easy enough to take off. As I stood there in front of Mohammed, I could not tell if he had any improvement in his vision. Stoic since our first meeting, his demeanor did not change. My heart began to sink as I asked the interpreter if Mohammed could see me. As he visually engaged me for the first time, Mohammed raised his arms and outstretched his long hands in glee. He excitedly raised his voice in his native language, and to this day I have never found out what he said. But I knew this was a good sign. I asked if he could count the fingers I held in front of my face. Better vision, but still legally blind. I then tested his visual acuity. As he progressively read the chart, from the 20/400 line, through 20/100, on down to finally read the 20/40 line on his first day after surgery, the emotional energy in the room was infectious. His wife and daughters were crying in delight, his advocate was amazed, my office staff (most were watching outside the room) were clapping, and I welled with joy too.

When Mohammed finally stood up, he reached out, clasped both my hands, looked me in the eye, and said, "Thank you." I could tell these were not words he spoke often, and I understood the significance of his gratefulness.

A week later, in a postoperative visit, Mohammed's vision had improved even further and he had a lightness to his personality that I had never seen before. Actually smiling and conversing, he clearly appreciated his new, better circumstances. We said our goodbyes and set up a final postop visit for three weeks later.

The next week, his advocate set up a lunchtime appointment with me and brought his young daughter— who had heard so much about Mohammed's saga that she wanted to meet his surgeon. The advocate told me that Mohammed and his family had moved to the East Coast, where he had found a job. He could stay in America! I wanted to keep in touch with him and his family but was told that would be impossible because no one from his church or Exodus World Service knew exactly where he was. I wanted to assure that he continue with his postop care to maintain the vision that was restored. It has been almost three years, but to this day I still worry about him. I think I always will.

Editor's Note: I first met Dr. Weiss when he was a medical student at Northwestern in Chicago. We worked together at the University of Chicago, where he trained in ophthalmology. He brings a human side to surgery, restoring sight to an immigrant, giving the patient a new chance at life.

What a Dog Can Teach a Cancer Surgeon about Death

Richard C. Karl, MD, FACS

O UR DOG, UBU, is dying. He's almost fifteen, a lab-
shepherd mix. We got him as a pup. He's been a
wonderful companion for all these years, and in the last
nine months he's taught me a lot about life and a little
about death. I work as a cancer surgeon, and matters of
death and dying are not altogether unfamiliar territory,
but I've learned a great deal more from watching the
changes in Ubu. The muscles in his head have atrophied
so that his skull is easily palpable just beneath his skin. He
can no longer walk. He doesn't bark anymore.

Hearing? He lost that a few years ago but was (back then) otherwise unbowed. Instead of asking him whether he'd enjoy a car ride, my wife learned to pantomime a driver's grip on the steering wheel. Once he saw that sign, he'd dart to the car, tail thumping, ears back. His natural exuberance has been a delight, though occasionally it has also been a distracting annoyance.

Like many dogs of his heritage, he was an enthusiastic, endlessly hopeful optimist. Any sign that a human being was heading to the refrigerator prompted his alert interest. All manner of conveyance pleased him. He'd sit in the back seat of the car, head out the window, his tongue dangling and a wake of saliva cascading onto the side of the vehicle. He loved boats, airplanes, and cars.

A powerful swimmer, Ubu loved going to several local "dog beaches," where he chased balls and sniffed the competition, but never did master the art of retrieval. He would swim out, apprehend the ball in his powerful jaws, turn, swim back to the shore, then, as his windmilling feet touched the bottom, he'd lose interest and drop the ball some four or five feet away from his masters as they hollered at him. Finally, we'd roll up our pants legs and wade out to retrieve the ball ourselves and start the whole dance over again.

He was not an undiscriminating dog. He had his preferences and he was true to them, whether they were his affection for broccoli or his dislike of one or two of our friends. He couldn't be bribed. He never ate to excess and was about 97 percent house trained. He possessed a noble sense of who he was. He had a point of view.

Then one night last year, we awoke to hear him thrashing in the house. It was three in the morning and he was in a room he rarely ventured into. When I got the lights on, he had a crazed look in his eye. He was seizing and incontinent. I hauled him into the back yard, laid him down, and tried to console him. He was not calmed. My wife, Cathy, came out, and the three of us lay in the grass, crying and naked. We were sure this was the end.

An hour later Ubu was breathing more easily and, after we cleaned him up, we brought him into the bedroom and took turns trying to sleep with him on the floor. Our dog did not die that night.

He had had a terrible stroke, I think. He could still walk, but his gait was unsteady and his movements were awkward. He kept turning his head to the left. He soon became less mobile and finally was unable to walk. I thought maybe he'd live a week or two, but that was nine months ago. He does not appear to be in pain, and he tracks our movements with his head and with his eyes. He has stabilized as a noble wounded creature.

"Should we put him to sleep?" We discuss this every day. When friends visit, they appear to group themselves into two camps. Some look uncertain, then finally wonder aloud as to whether he wouldn't be better off dead. Others seem to support what we're doing. They talk about a "natural death" with reverence and care. When I think about the natural death of an animal, though, I think of a dog going off somewhere to die peacefully. Ubu's incapacitation is such that he can't do this. We're not supporting him with a feeding tube or a respirator, but he wouldn't survive if we didn't bring him his food and water and keep him clean. He could stop eating, but he hasn't.

Sometimes I see an interesting thing in the patients I serve. When a patient and her spouse are close, still in love with each other, a curious argument sometimes comes to light. The patient, knowing she has recurrent breast cancer, say, wants to have good, quality time with her husband. The husband, knowing how bereft he'll feel when she's gone, wants her to endure any therapy so as to keep her alive as long as possible, even though the quality of that longer life may be poor. It is a sweet tactical argument, really. They love each other but see the end of life differently. One wants quality and the other wants length. When it comes to Ubu, we seem to be in the length camp.

Are we being selfish by keeping our dog fed and watered? Would I want the same treatment? I often tell Cathy that with Ubu she is practicing for me. I am kidding, but only slightly. I know that the renowned Washington columnist Mary McGrory said to a close friend after she had a stroke, "It is worse than death." It took all her energy to make that one simple statement. I have the sense that I'd like to keep living if I've got the support and still enjoy a little steak and potatoes, but today I am not at that point, and I won't know my feelings for sure until I *do* reach that point.

We went to see Dr. Arthur Caplan, a well-known ethicist from the University of Pennsylvania, when he came to town a couple of weeks ago. He talked about the "persistent vegetative state," as well as Karen Ann Quinlan and Terry Schiavo. He implored his audience to have living wills and advance directives, surrogate healthcare decision makers and a clear understanding with doctors. He didn't help me with the sixty-five canine pounds of appetite that I have at my feet right now. Dogs don't talk, make living wills, or have much use for lawyers—unless they bite somebody.

I met a young woman who seemed taken aback when I told her about Ubu. She has two golden retrievers, each weighing ninety pounds or more. I know she loves dogs in general and her own in particular. She did tell me that she had them in "doggie day care" two days a week. "I know they love the social aspects, and I feel better when I get home from work and am too tired to take them for a run," she told me. I said to her, "If you had told me this five years ago, I would have laughed. Now I know that we do things for our dogs that can be hard for others to understand."

Are pets surrogates for the close human bonds that we seek often and find infrequently? Some posit so. I know that our dog is not in a persistent vegetative state. I know that he loves to peel and eat shrimp. I know that my wife and I have stopped planning trips together, as one of us needs to be here all the time. This does not feel burdensome. When I see a healthy, active dog, I am drawn to him. I am reminded of a satisfying relationship with another living creature; it is a good memory.

This morning when I got up, Ubu had his head up.

He devoured some salmon, and his eyes were luminous. I asked him one more time if I was doing the right thing for him. He looked at me with those beautiful brown eyes, licked his lips, and had a sip of water. I feel forgiven.

Editor's Note: Dr. Karl was the Chairman of Surgery at the University of South Florida and the Director of the Division of Surgical Oncology. As one who owns four basset hounds and has three family members with cancer, I was touched on many levels by this story and its unusual perspective.

Not a Hired Gun

Arthur W. Perry, MD, FACS

I SUPPOSE IT WAS Aaron who turned me into a medical conservative. And I'm not talking politics.

On the day I began my plastic surgery residency at the University of Chicago, Aaron was a rotund sixty-seven-year-old diabetic patient in the intensive care unit. He was recovering from necrotizing fasciitis, the rare "flesh-eating" disease that is so frightening that an Internet search reveals more than 241,000 stories about it. Aaron's disease started with a pimple on his scrotum. With his immune system crippled by sky-high blood sugar levels, bacteria from the pimple grazed on his tissue like sheep munching on grass. His infection spread and, by the time he showed up in the emergency room, had encompassed his penis, scrotum, thighs, and lower abdomen. By the time I met him, he had already survived two trips to the operating room to remove dead infected tissue and replace it with skin grafted from his outer thighs. Aaron was moved out of intensive care to a regular hospital floor, where he spent the next few weeks healing and gaining strength. He was discharged from the hospital on a sunny day in July, sans penis and testicles.

Every two weeks, like clockwork, Aaron showed up at the residents' clinic where I charted the progress of his recovery. And every visit, never missing one, Aaron asked to have his penis reconstructed. After a year and half, with his terrifying illness long behind him and his diabetes well controlled, his insistence to have a new penis created was becoming stronger. We had all rolled our eyes at Aaron's requests, but he wore us down and eventually we gave in. A surgical date was scheduled. At the time, I thought it was odd that a sixty-seven-year-old man would care so much about his penis, but the 25 million men who use Viagra answered that question two decades later.

A team consisting of an attending plastic surgeon, four residents, and the usual crew of wide-eyed medical students and nurses all helped create a spectacular-looking penis for Aaron—one worthy of publication. We took the tissue from his forearm and wrapped skin, a little muscle, and even a bone for rigidity into a penis that looked as real as any (in the dark, anyway). We microsurgically connected arteries, veins, and even nerves that would eventually supply sensation. After ten hours in the operating room, the exhausted team wheeled Aaron into the recovery room. In his semiprivate room the next morning, Aaron and the team marveled over his new penis. I can't even imagine what his roommate was thinking.

As the days progressed, his stitches and drains were removed, all wounds had healed, and Aaron was ready for discharge. One last walk around the floor satisfied the physical therapist that Aaron would be safe at home. As Aaron hopped back into bed, thrilled to be going home, the nurse noticed a little blood on his gown and requested that I check him out before discharge. To my horror, Aaron's new penis was pale, meaning that the microsurgical connections had failed; we needed a rapid return to the operating room to reattach the vessels and salvage the reconstruction. While failures in microsurgery are most common in the first two days after surgery, Aaron had managed to detach the blood vessels nearly two weeks after surgery.

Within an hour, Aaron was under general anesthesia, and the incision was made. The blood vessels were in plain view, stretched and clotted but intact. Our first move before embarking on a time-consuming disassembly and reassembly of the junctions of the arteries and veins was to inject the obstruction with the clot-buster streptokinase. Bacteria manufacture this chemical, much the same way penicillin is produced, for the benefit of humans. Streptokinase is an enzyme that can chew right through blood clots, clearing blood vessels. It's so potent that it can reverse heart attacks and strokes. And so, with the words "Bombs away," the attending surgeon injected the streptokinase. We waited for the clot to clear. No effect, but sometimes a higher dose is needed. As we readied to inject more, the anesthesiologist yelled to us to stop surgery. Aaron's heart had slowed. Immediately after injection of the streptokinase, he had the most severe type of allergic reaction, called anaphylaxis. Steroids and epinephrine were pumped through Aaron's intravenous lines, but his heart stopped. Frantic pumps on his chest were tried, followed by 360 joules of pure energy delivered by a defibrillator. After forty-five minutes of resuscitation, the code was stopped. Aaron had died.

Surgeons do not take death lightly. There are some fields, like cardiac and burn surgery, where death is unfortunately not uncommon. But death is not supposed to happen in plastic surgery. Plastic surgeons reconstruct people. We make them look better. It was incomprehensible that Aaron had survived a devastating infection and severe diabetes but died trying to obtain a new penis. Aaron's death taught me a lot about life, about surgery, and about my responsibility to patients. Medical ethicists can argue about whether a sixty-seven-year-old man should have his penis reconstructed, and some might extend that argument to *any* procedure with *any* risk in anyone with *any* illness. Some could argue that no cosmetic surgery should ever be performed, because it is not lifesaving and has no medical benefit. Aaron could still urinate without a penis, and he would never be able to perform sexually even with a reconstructed one. Other ethicists might say that the patient should make an informed decision and it would be arrogant for the surgeon to oppose it.

Attempts at surgery hundreds of years ago were extremely dangerous. The development of anesthesia in the nineteenth century allowed surgery to be performed without unbearable pain. The best surgeons of the Civil War era were the ones who could cut off a leg the fastest, shortening the duration of the patient's unbearable pain, using only Jim Beam as an anesthetic. Antibiotics revolutionized surgery in the 1940s, but only in the last three decades have invasive operations had unprecedented safety. The death rate from general anesthesia has decreased from one in two thousand in 1980 to one in half a million now. This miraculous change is largely due to better monitors and safer drugs.

But surgery still has its risks, and Aaron's death drilled that fact into my psyche. Aaron was the last patient I operated on who died in the operating room. With my practice now restricted to cosmetic surgery, I believe that this type of surgery should only be performed on healthy patients, a philosophy that is clearly discriminatory against disease but not against people. My patients need to be cleared by internists before I agree to operate on them; and even *with* clearance, sometimes I need to be convinced that the surgery will be safe. I have turned down overweight people who wanted liposuction, men with heart disease who wanted face-lifts, and women with previous blood clots in their legs who wanted tummy tucks. Many of these people eventually went to other plastic surgeons who, unfortunately, performed their surgery, sometimes with unfavorable outcomes.

Unfortunately, patients with full wallets will always find a willing surgeon eventually.

For more than three decades I have listened to doctors present their complications at monthly conferences at the medical schools with which I've been affiliated. And for more than ten years I sat in judgment of other doctors as the governor's appointee to the New Jersey State Board of Medical Examiners. All the complaints about surgeons came before me. I listened over and over to complaints about doctors, many of the charges triggered by bad outcomes—complications and deaths. Frequently I found a reason for the complication—too much fat removed (death), not stopping birth control pills (blood clots in the legs), and poor lung function (pneumonia). In a perfect world, there would be no complications. But even if every little detail in patient care is perfectly performed, a certain percentage of patients will still have a complication. There's no physical way to completely eliminate infection, for instance. There's just no way around it. But when I listen to doctors say things like, "We get away with it most of the time," I get a chill down my spine, knowing that what they're really saying is "The procedure is not uniformly safe, but we can usually pull it off." Or, after a complication, a surgeon will say, "He was cleared by cardiology for the procedure" and feel exonerated after a bad outcome. But sometimes internists don't understand that their standard for "surgical clearance" needs to be higher for cosmetic surgery than for a gallbladder removal.

My attitude is that cosmetic surgery should be uniformly safe, or at least as safe as humanly possible. Risks that are justified for procedures that treat disease are not acceptable in cosmetic surgery. Diabetics need to have their festering appendix out or they will face certain death. And they might need a hip replacement or they'll be in a wheelchair. But they don't need face-lifts or liposuction.

Plastic surgeons have a responsibility to keep patients safe. And sometimes that means they need to protect patients from themselves. Often, patients who have high risks for surgical complications tell me they are willing to accept the risks, are willing even to sign a paper discharging my liability if something bad happens. But like a financial adviser with a fiduciary responsibility to protect a client's fortune, or a parent with responsibility to keep children safe, a plastic surgeon is not a hired gun, ready to do any requested task. Few surgeons would comply with a patient requesting amputation of a perfectly good thumb. The patient might be doing it for cosmetic reasons—better symmetry of the hand, perhaps. I believe it is likewise unethical to perform a procedure that has high risks when undertaken simply to improve appearance.

Of course, there's a gray line somewhere that ethicists like to discuss. What exactly defines high risk? Where do we draw the line: is hypertension and a family history of heart disease enough to exclude a patient from an eyelid lift? Few surgeons would think so. But that patient does have a higher chance of a complication after surgery. And so a thoughtful surgeon might obtain a cardiology consult and perform a stress test to bring the risks back down to acceptable levels.

And then there's the question of what level of deformity crosses the line from simply cosmetic to psychologically injurious. When does a large nose become a deformity and justify higher risk? What degree of breast asymmetry is normal and what interferes with proper psychological development? These are the questions that require both common sense and sound surgical judgment. And they cannot be easily answered.

When patients come to me, they choose me and I choose them. They need to feel comfortable with my skills and personality, and I need to know they are appropriate candidates for surgery—medically and psychologically. Aaron is always with me, protecting my patients from operating on them unnecessarily.

THE MELANOMA

James S. Goydos, MD, FACS

ONE OF THE most important decisions a physician makes is whether to specialize or become a generalist. Surgeons make this decision after their initial general surgical training, and it profoundly affects the course of not only their careers but also their home life and even their daily mood. I decided, after five long years of general surgical training, to pursue a career as a surgical oncologist, a surgeon who treats patients with cancer.

Surgical oncology training, which takes an additional two to three years after a five-year residency, is known as a tough fellowship. Not only are there typically long hours of work and psychologically difficult situations dealing with patients with devastating diseases, but there are technically complex operations to master. While in my fellowship at the University of Pittsburgh School of Medicine, I had the privilege of working with some of the most skilled surgeons in the country. Their knowledge and skills rubbed off on me, and at the end of my training I decided that I would be a *hepatobiliary* surgeon. That's a word most people have never even heard of; it means working on liver, pancreas, and bile duct tumors, dealing with intricate anatomy and some of the most complex operations in all of medicine.

By the time I had completed my fellowship, my wife had already finished her own fellowship—in high-risk obstetrics—and had taken a job with her old boss at the Robert Wood Johnson Medical School in New Jersey. Most people don't realize that the more highly specialized the physician, the fewer job opportunities there are. Geographically, I was limited to a handful of employment opportunities, and as life would have it, the year I completed my training was also the year that no jobs for an aspiring liver surgeon were available within close enough range to my wife so that we could still have a normal family life.

But my calling card was the internationally known program I had just completed at the University of Pittsburgh. Pitt was famous for treating not only hepatobiliary cancers but also the skin cancer known as melanoma. Melanomas are those pigmented skin cancers that are notorious for spreading to the lungs, liver, and brain, often killing patients within a few years. But they are interesting tumors, with an unusual biology—sometimes returning after decades and sometimes being cured despite widespread disease. During an interview at the Cancer Institute of New Jersey, I was told that the liver surgery program was well staffed but that they needed a melanoma surgeon. Desperate to stay in New Jersey, I took the melanoma position and began to build a program.

While not my first choice of a career, melanoma is a fascinating disease, ripe for a surgeon with an inquisitive mind. I had to admit that I did fit the bill. Over the next decade I built one of the largest melanoma programs in the northeastern United States, but I was never completely satisfied with my career choice. Like a 747-trained pilot who was relegated to flying propeller planes between New York and Philadelphia, I was haunted by a continuing desire to be a liver surgeon. Those were the guys who performed the most complex and difficult operations. They were the most respected of the surgical oncologists—not exactly the reputation of melanoma surgeons. Other surgeons regarded the melanoma guys as just "skin doctors." Did I really spend more than a decade of surgical training to become a "skin doctor"?

Melanoma is a complex disease that requires a caring, thinking, but aggressive surgeon to save the patients' lives. But that's not enough; the surgeon must be a masterful technician, performing operations that are varied and often complex. Nevertheless, melanoma surgeons lack respect from other surgeons. And quite frankly, they don't have the mystique of cardiac or neurosurgeons—or the glamour of plastic surgeons. Melanoma surgeons are like the utility players in the major leagues: ready for any situation but never getting on the cover of *Sports Illustrated*.

Then, seven years after arriving in New Jersey, I met Maria, a patient who changed my perspective forever. Maria was a sixtysomething-year-old Hispanic woman who went to the emergency room with belly pain and a feeling of weakness. Her blood count turned out to be very low, and then her doctor found the cause of her problem. She had a mass in her esophagus, the tube that connects the mouth with the stomach. A scope was passed down Maria's esophagus, and a piece of the lump was sent to the pathologists to look at under the microscope. Maria's doctors expected to find an esophageal cancer, but to their surprise the lump turned out to be a melanoma—a skin cancer in the esophagus!

And now the mystery. Here was a patient with no known melanoma on her skin but a cancer somehow spread to her esophagus. She apparently had what doctors call "mets," short for *metastases*. Her doctors surmised that sometime in the previous few years, cells broke off from a tiny skin cancer, traveled through her blood, and set up shop in her esophagus. And then they grew. Metastatic melanoma kills almost 100 percent of the time, so the news couldn't have been worse for Maria. But it did get worse. Maria's heart wasn't strong enough to tolerate the chemotherapy that her doctors thought she needed. She and her family were told that nothing could be done, and Maria was offered hospice care and pain medications to make her comfortable.

Most of the family resigned themselves to the inevitable, but Maria's oldest daughter wasn't ready to give up. She contacted medical oncologists around the state, who all gave her the same answer: her mother wouldn't be able to tolerate the needed chemotherapy. She was also told that her mother's disease was so severe that chemotherapy would probably not be useful. Still that didn't stop her. Maria's daughter called me at the end of a busy day and pleaded for me to help her mother. At first thought, I agreed with Maria's other doctors, but something in her story didn't sound quite right. Maria was a Hispanic woman with dark skin pigmentation and no history of a melanoma of her skin. Melanoma is rare in dark-skinned individuals, and it is even rarer to not have an obvious spot on the skin. My curiosity was piqued. I asked her daughter to bring Maria in to see me in my clinic the following Monday.

It is never a good situation when a patient is brought to an appointment on a stretcher by an ambulance crew. And sure enough, Maria was weak, frail, and in obvious pain. But it was fortunate for Maria that her daughter hadn't given up. I examined Maria and looked at a pile of x-rays and scans. And then it hit me. Maria didn't have skin cancer after all. Maria had a skin cancer that wasn't a skin cancer. Her type of melanoma was less likely to occur than an asteroid hitting downtown Los Angeles. Maria's melanoma hadn't *traveled* to her esophagus—it started there!

If I was correct, the thing to do was to remove the diseased section of the esophagus, which is an enormous and complex operation. I convinced the family and my colleagues that this was the proper course of action, and we operated on Maria the following week. The surgery was difficult, but we brought a skilled team to the table and were able to remove the entire tumor and surrounding lymph nodes despite her weakened condition. As I helped wheel her to the intensive care unit, I thought about Maria and I thought about my chosen career. If you can imagine how nice it feels to do a favor for another person and multiply that by ten thousand, you can begin to understand how I felt after operating on Maria.

Almost immediately after her operation, Maria began to feel better. The first taste of food that she swallowed without pain brought a feeble smile to her face. She gained strength each day and was discharged from the hospital less than two weeks after her marathon procedure. Two weeks after her discharge she saw me in the outpatient clinic. She was still weak, but I will remember her smile for the rest of my life. I followed her for almost five years, and her cancer never came back.

I will likely never know for sure whether her melanoma originated in her esophagus. But I do know that if I hadn't considered one of the rarest of all possibilities, I would have never cured her of her disease. If it had been spread from her skin, then there would have been microscopic disease throughout her body that would have killed her long ago.

A year ago I received a card in the mail from the patient's daughter. Maria had died the week before—not of melanoma, but of heart disease—six years after I operated on her "fatal" disease. Her daughter thanked me for allowing Maria to see the college graduation of her granddaughter, the first family member ever to reach that milestone. As I put the card down, I smiled to myself. Maybe mystique is overrated and it isn't so bad being a "skin doctor" after all.

Editor's Note: Dr. Goydos is known as one of the smartest surgeons at Robert Wood Johnson; I've even had him remove a mole from me. This story ties in with Dr. Silen's story; a good surgeon must be a thinking physician first, a technician second.

A Detour

Bruce L. Gewertz, MD, FACS

L IKE SO MANY of my colleagues, I emerged from four years of medical school a bit surprised that despite the parade of "classic" symptoms that I experienced (rabies and the plague were among my many imaginary maladies), I had miraculously escaped premature death from the diseases I studied. As I grew older and became a vascular surgeon, I developed a strong tendency to deny or trivialize any personal complaints or physical findings. This attitude notably differed from the alarmist mentality I had embraced as a young man and, best of all, further separated me from the "worried well" who gravitated to me at cocktail parties and my medical office. I eschewed regular physical examinations and complied only begrudgingly with highly specific preventive maintenance such as colonoscopies and prostate-specific ambigen (PSA) measurements. I had my elevated blood pressure measured on occasion and literally "took my medicine" reliably and with some amusement.

In November of 2007 I noted a discoid thickening under my left nipple. I knew that the blood pressure medicine I took sometimes caused such breast changes, even in men, and was not alarmed. Still, there really was something there—every time I looked for it—and unlike other lumps and bumps, it did not just go away. In January I consulted a trusted colleague. Owing to the informality of my approach, it was hardly a doctor's visit; more like a typical "curbside consult" in his office late one Friday afternoon. He felt my lump, reassured me that gynecomastia from drugs was the most likely cause, yet clearly recommended that he remove it. We just had to pick the right date so it wouldn't interfere with my golf and work schedule.

Over the next several months, my hectic schedule as surgeon in chief of the Cedars-Sinai Medical Center in Los Angeles never quite allowed me to act on his recommendation. Moreover, the lump never changed in size. I congratulated myself for my good judgment in avoiding a needless procedure. After all, when surgeons are asked to fill in the blank after "Surgery is," we are known to say, "Surgery is for other people."

One day in April 2008, I was drying off after a shower in the gym and couldn't help but see that things had definitely changed; my left nipple was pinched in and markedly distorted. I knew immediately from my earlier general surgery training that this was a clear sign of cancer. I telephoned my colleague, who was at a medical meeting out of town. With one call, he arranged for a mammogram and ultrasound the next morning. It was the first of many times in my illness that my professional status gave me extraordinary access to timely care.

The mammogram and ultrasound were followed within an hour by a biopsy, which confirmed cancer. Although the diagnosis was expected, the words had real emotional impact. Still, it was a perfect Southern California spring afternoon and I couldn't mourn. The prognosis was good if not perfect, and either way there would be many more fine days. A friend met me for lunch. We commiserated over both of our health challenges; we admired the beautiful waitresses. Beer was consumed.

I had a professional commitment to a close friend to give an Honor Society lecture in Florida that weekend. Ironically, my topic was "finding balance in your personal and professional life." I soldiered on, since a late cancellation would have been a major letdown and my surgery wasn't scheduled for a few days. To be sure, my "personal life balance" wasn't perfect; unfairly, my loving wife was left at home to think alone while I was pleasantly distracted by seeing my good friends and doing my duty.

The cross-country flights allowed more than enough time for reflection; the altitude and spectacular sunset seemed an obvious invitation to gain a broader perspective. On the way east, I processed the implications of the pathology report; on the way west, I steeled myself for the surgery later that day. The flight attendant never quite figured out I was "nothing by mouth—preop" and endlessly proffered food and wine. I was taken into the operating room less than two hours after landing in L.A. When I awoke, my friend and surgeon reassured me that things looked good; the breast was removed and my "sentinel" lymph nodes, the closest ones to the tumor, were clean.

I had little pain after surgery, thanks to the expertise of my colleagues and the euphoria of a good outcome. I missed two workdays and figured the episode was behind me. Unfortunately, when the pathology report showed an aggressive tumor just under two centimeters in size, it was clear that chemotherapy and radiation would likely be recommended.

I was referred to an oncologist. Rather than see me in her office, she insisted that she visit me in mine. At the end of her long day, she spent more than an hour going over the decision making and rationale for chemo. As she went to leave, she embraced me. For the first of many times, a physician's kindness and dedication were nearly overwhelming to me.

Given my visibility at the hospital, I needed to make things public. After all, I certainly intended to work, even if I might not operate, and it would be hard to fake losing my hair. Email was an effective route. I sent this message out to my colleagues:

I wanted to keep you up to date on my personal medical situation. I underwent a left mastectomy and sentinel node dissection 2 weeks ago for breast cancer. The node was negative implying a very good prognosis (T1 No). I have fully recovered from the procedure. Seeing the hospital from a different perspective was actually quite gratifying; the care and kindness were extraordinary. I am very proud to work here.

That said, despite the favorable outlook, my physician is likely going to recommend adjuvant (prophylactic) chemotherapy and radiation. She assures me that absent complications, I should be able to work nearly a normal schedule during the four months of treatment, apparently sans hair. I have canceled all travel plans and taken a leave from most outside obligations; this will allow me to concentrate fully on my work here and my health.

I appreciate your kind words and help during this time. I am confident that we can continue to do great things together in the upcoming years.

Chemotherapy began and (mercifully) ended three months later, with much misery in between. After a brief respite, I began two months of radiation treatments under the attentive care of a wonderful radiation oncologist and her team. They were unfailingly upbeat and were implausibly happy to see me every day at 2 P.M. for so many afternoons. Slowly, very slowly, I regained energy.

By Thanksgiving, I was finally able to walk more than a hundred feet at a time and could accompany my wife and dog on beautiful weekend walks—a far cry from my usual ninety-minute workouts, but a blessing nonetheless.

Despite the physical suffering, it was remarkable how so much of what I experienced was positive. First and foremost, you never know how your partner will respond to your serious illness. Previously, I was rarely sick in our years together, and when I was, always a surgical type, I tended to get a few liters of fluid infused intravenously and head back to work. In this challenge, that wouldn't be nearly enough. I needed my wife's support, and it was unfailing. She would follow my lead, minimizing introspection but dealing practically with each issue as it came up. When my hair started coming out in clumps (unfortunately beginning at our friends' cabin in New Hampshire), we both laughed as she shaved my head in the backyard; the New Age look would have to do for a while. At least in my presence, she left out the feeling sorry part but told me she loved me every day. Before my illness, I had had no reason to doubt her steadfast character; still, it was now beautifully revealed for anyone to see, and it made our relationship even stronger.

Support from family and friends was uniform, it and made all the difference. Our children, widely distributed across the country, called daily. My parents thoughtfully visited when I was up for it. There was not a day that went by without emails or calls from my friends, letting me know I was in their thoughts. I arrived for work one day to find two of my colleagues had shaved their own heads in sympathy (although to be historically accurate, one had little hair to lose!). Friends and their children dedicated charity bike rides to me. As I viewed the pictures of their enthusiastic efforts or read the letters and emails, it was a revelation to me how much joy each act of kindness and expression of concern brought to me. Indeed, even when I didn't leave the house for a week, I never felt more connected. I vowed to remember and pass the feeling on in the future.

Work was a sustaining factor. Whether I was working from home or in my office, no matter how challenging the problem was, dealing with it made me feel productive and vital. My executive assistant became a fierce protector and advocate, taking on a vast range of tasks and allowing me to marshal my resources for the critical issues that needed my input. As I walked the halls, the expressions of goodwill were priceless reminders that I had not dropped off anyone's radar.

In my interactions with my doctors, there was no question I thought and felt like the patient I was, not an experienced physician. I was aided in this role reversal by the fact that treatment of breast cancer has been totally revolutionized since my general surgical training more than thirty years ago. I asked more than a few questions, always preferring to get the answers from my physicians rather than to search my library or the Internet. After all, these would be the opinions of people I had chosen, who knew me and the particulars of my case. In fact, when offered reading materials on the subject, I tended to disregard the articles and simply to ask what my doctor thought was best.

Of all the insights I gained in the professional arena, none was more important than the degree to which words and numbers are perceived differently by patient and doctor. As a doctor, when I told patients they had a 90 percent chance of surviving ten years, I felt I was giving them great news. As a patient, it sounded just short of grim. I found myself listening for every nuance in physicians' comments. Months after my treatment ended, a well-meaning gastroenterologist said he would do another screening colonoscopy in five years "if we are both still around." It wasn't funny and bothers me still.

I have been a student of the positive effects of optimism in medicine, sports, and life. I frequently point out to our surgical trainees the clear evidence that your attitude influences your ability to perform in the operating room as well as your survival from illness or surgery. That said, for perhaps the first time in my life, I felt doubt that I would be around at seventy-five. I have come to believe that this was a strange type of defensive and fatalistic reaction. I just wanted to be sure I wasn't devastated emotionally if the cancer returned.

I have since regrouped. Acknowledging that nothing is guaranteed to any of us, I now take time each day to take stock of the great opportunities I have been given to do good things. I renew my determination to overcome those few misguided cells that sent me on this detour and daily convince myself that there is much I can and will do to keep playing.

Editor's Note: Bruce Gewertz, the Chairman of Surgery at Cedar-Sinai Medical Center in Los Angeles, tells his personal story of how he, a man, developed breast cancer. Doctors often feel that illness "is for other people" and when it strikes home, they react differently than non-medical people. Dr. Gewertz, who played himself, and was the technical advisor, in the movie The Fugitive *and I were together at the University of Chicago.*

A Diagnostic Dilemma

Jane E. Miller, MD, FACOG

I'M A GYNECOLOGIST. Not an everyday gynecologist, but the kind that helps infertile women become pregnant. It's a relatively new specialty—a mix of reproductive endocrinology, gynecology, surgery, and a little luck. Put all those together, add what we call in vitro fertilization (IVF), and I help women who can't get pregnant on their own have a baby.

Alicia and her husband had been trying to get pregnant for three years and I was their third stop. They were both thirty-seven and she had never been pregnant. They braved two bridges and New York traffic to get to my New Jersey office. Had I been the patient, I would have hired a bellhop to carry those thick stacks of old records from past tries, but she was five-ten, 186 pounds, and, as is so often said in medical parlance, "otherwise within normal limits." She deposited the files on my desk.

Alicia's prior workup had been routine, and she had undergone several unsuccessful fertility treatment cycles. She had predictable monthly periods and a normal hormonal panel, and all her husband's semen analysis was normal as well. There was only one thing in her history that, perhaps, was a clue to her infertility: her periods were getting more and more painful every month. Pain with periods is not uncommon and usually diminishes as a woman ages. Alicia's was worsening, and despite her "high threshold for pain" she sometimes missed work, stayed in bed, and consumed more Advil than the recommended daily dose. One of her previous doctors had performed a laparoscopy in which he used a small telescope to look inside her pelvis. He had discovered endometriosis (a disease that can cause painful periods), but it was so minimal that he had told her "not to worry." In endometriosis, the tissue that normally lines the inside of the uterus grows in other areas inside the abdomen. The more endometriosis she has, the less likely a woman is to become pregnant. I concluded my history taking with two notes scribbled in the margins of the chart: increased age and rule out active endometriosis.

When I examined her, I discovered an abdomen that was so distended and tense that it rendered my pelvic exam worthless. I could not feel her uterus or ovaries. I asked her if she had gained weight or noticed any recent change in her appetite, bowel activity, or energy.

"Yeah, my jeans are a little tight just when I take them out of the dryer," she answered. Darn stretch jeans; they can adapt to anything! Alicia obviously didn't know that there was a problem. I didn't want to alarm her, but I was concerned. I needed to do some important tests to make sure she didn't have a serious problem.

I performed a vaginal sonogram to image her uterus and ovaries, but to my surprise, these organs were not to be found. All that could be seen was massive ascites, fluid inside the abdomen and pelvis, and the occasional loop of bowel floating in this ocean of fluid. I explained to Alicia that the fertility testing that we had begun would be done in conjunction with an investigation of the ascites. I did not tell her that I was worried that she might have ovarian cancer.

My attempt to perform an x-ray of the inside of her uterus and tubes was useless. Contrast is injected through the cervix into the uterus in this test and pictures are taken. In fertility lingo it is called an HSG or, in lay terms, "the dye test." But Alicia's cervix was in such an abnormal position that I could not place a catheter within it. That same day she walked off the MRI table, claiming claustrophobia. To top it off, she was disgusted. "I came to you to get pregnant, Dr. Miller," she said. "I don't want all this." "You can't get pregnant like this," I told her. "You can't *be* pregnant like this! Please hang in there!" She agreed to a CT scan.

On CT scan, she had massive ascites but her ovaries appeared normal. I wasn't any further ahead than when I had done my own sonogram. I sent off a battery of blood tests and found that Alicia's CA125, called the "ovarian cancer test," was markedly elevated. I knew that other diseases might also cause an abnormal number, but an elevated CA125 in the presence of massive ascites almost clinched the dreaded diagnosis of ovarian cancer. It was time to examine the fluid.

With ease (and a little sedation) I put a needle through her vagina into her pelvis and drew off a couple of ounces of fluid. If tumor cells were present, the lab would identify them. I expected the ascites to be cloudy white or golden in color but what I obtained was dark brown. The pathologist did not find any evidence of malignancy. Great news—but what was causing the ascites?

Dark ascites is usually not something seen by reproductive endocrinologists like myself. But I remembered a lecture in medical school thirty years earlier that had described a patient with just that. I picked up the phone and called my father. Dad was eighty-eight at the time, retired from private practice and part-time teaching of pulmonary and internal medicine at the State University of New York Downstate College of Medicine. The rumor spread by the residents and fellows there was that Dr. Hy Miller was so smart that he had memorized Harrison's textbook of internal medicine and could quote, verbatim, from every page. In his day he had treated some of the greats: Louis Armstrong and Howard Cosell, among others. He was one of the first doctors to use penicillin. He had done some of the groundbreaking work on asbestos and lung disease. I presented the case to him. "Budd-

Chiari syndrome," he said. "Obstruction of the hepatic vein," the big vein that drains the liver.

I went back and reviewed old texts and newer literature online. The syndrome affects one in a hundred thousand people, usually women, and can lead to cirrhosis and liver failure. And only two-thirds of patients live for more than ten years after the diagnosis. Pregnancy was no longer an issue. It was time to refer the patient for definitive diagnosis and treatment.

I sent Alicia to a well-known cancer surgeon who had extensive experience with liver disease. But he was convinced that she had a gynecologic malignancy, so he sent her to a gynecologic oncologic surgeon, who in turn was convinced that she did not have a gynecologic malignancy and sent her back to me. Once again I was no further along than I had been when I had first discovered the ascites. It was time to look inside Alicia's belly with a laparoscopy.

But with all that fluid in the way, how was I going to put a quarter-inch-diameter telescope through her navel and into her pelvis and expect to see anything? I convinced Alicia to allow me to remove the fluid in my office the day before surgery, and with the help of my anesthesiologist and a big egg retrieval needle, I drained *two and a half gallons* of fluid from her pelvis and abdomen. This fluid, however, was not dark brown as it had been before but reddish brown, and it tested positive for blood. Alicia had begun her period two days before: this fluid was probably menstrual fluid that had flowed backward through her fallopian tubes and into her pelvis. I wondered if this could explain her endometriosis, since backward menstrual flow was one of the theories of how it occurs. And so it was off to the operating room the next day. As I inserted the scope into her pelvis, indeed I found a very nasty case of endometriosis, complete with blue-black and red nodules, and scar tissue between the surfaces of her organs.

Endometriosis with ascites, that large amount of fluid we found in her belly, is unusual: there have been only thirty cases reported in the world. We worry about cancer when we see ascites; now we were free from that concern and could consider, again, the issue of pregnancy.

If the ascites was caused by Alicia's endometriosis, I had to figure out how to keep the disease at bay while I was treating her to get pregnant. But any treatment for endometriosis would preclude pregnancy, and any treatment for pregnancy would stimulate the growth of endometriosis and her ascites.

Over the next three months I gave Alicia monthly injections of Lupron to control the endometriosis, and sure enough, the ascites did not return. With the fluid gone and her pelvic organs back in their normal position, I was now able to do the x-ray test to image the inside of her uterus. I found a fibroid, a benign growth which would leave no room for an embryo to implant and grow. So we returned to the hospital OR, where I removed the fibroid and installed a balloon catheter in the uterus to keep its walls from sticking together while it healed.

"And now," I addressed Alicia and her husband one afternoon back in my office, "we are ready to talk pregnancy."

After a patient is treated for endometriosis, she is, in a sense, on a time clock—she must take advantage of a certain window of opportunity. If the patient is left to attempt pregnancy on her own, the disease can return within a year. In Alicia's case, however, once the Lupron injections were stopped her ascites would return. Worse, endometriosis can injure a woman's eggs. Given her complex history, Alicia's chances of conceiving and successfully completing a pregnancy with her own eggs was probably less than 10 percent. For these reasons I suggested using donated eggs and her husband's sperm. To my relief the couple was on board.

Carol, our egg donor coordinator, always makes the perfect donor-recipient matches. Together we pored over our files of screened donor photographs and profiles, searching for someone who was around five-ten and who had Alicia's features and coloring. No one seemed appropriate. "Don't worry. I'll find the right person," Carol said as she ran out the door, late for her own eye-doctor appointment. This appointment could not have been better timed: a newly hired receptionist who looked uncannily like Alicia greeted Carol when she arrived for her eye exam. Carol briefly explained what we were searching for and the woman agreed to come to our office to begin the donor screening process. Within three weeks Alicia and her donor were matched.

My remaining task was to stimulate the development of multiple eggs in the ovaries of the donor and, at the same time, prepare Alicia's uterine lining to receive embryos. This is a routine procedure in which egg donors and recipients are "cycled" together, but Alicia's case once again posed a problem. The hormonal treatment required to develop her uterine lining would, for about two weeks, allow the ascites to begin to reaccumulate. If she were to get pregnant from the embryo transfer, the endometriosis would be stifled and she would be fine. If the IVF did not work, in several months' time she would have accumulated fluid and, once again, would have painful periods. It was like a double jeopardy—a scene from a movie. I presented the possible scenarios to Alicia and her husband. "We've come this far, Dr. Miller. We don't want to stop now," they said together. I opened the window.

Alicia's pregnancy, like any other, had its challenges, but at term she delivered a healthy girl and boy. She came to see me six months later, family in tow and an abdomen once again full of fluid but with the biggest smile on her face. "We'll get through this, Dr. Miller," she said this time.

Alicia comes to see me once a month. She still braves two bridges and New York traffic to get to my office. In fact, her car could probably get here by itself without her driving it. But there is no more ascites and she is not in pain. In fact, everything is just fine.

Editor's Note: Many people do not often think of gynecologists when they think of surgeons. However, gynecologists do perform a wide variety of surgery. I first met Dr. Miller when we were both residents at Harvard. Her amazing skills have created babies for countless women.

THE SURGERY OF SNEETCHES

Thomas J. Krizek, MD, FACS

Now, the Star-Belly Sneetches
Had bellies with stars.
The Plain-Belly Sneetches
Had none upon thars.
... Dr. Seuss, *The Sneetches and Other Stories*

AND THUSLY DID Dr. Seuss capture the essence of what plastic (and reconstructive) surgery meant to me during my thirty-five years in the field. In the Sneetch world, those with stars on their bellies thought they were better and bragged, "We're the best kind of Sneetch on the beach." The star-bellied Sneetches looked down on and meaningfully excluded those Sneetches without stars. Some in our society, like the Sneetches, are fortunate enough to have a "normal" if not "beautiful" appearance; they have the metaphorical equivalent of "stars" on their bellies. Others, many of whom became our patients, are less fortunate and are either born without stars or, through injury, cancer, or even normal aging, lose the stars that they once had. I have been privileged to be one of those who, through a combination of art and science, can help provide these missing stars.

To Dr. Seuss's Sneetches, these stars were an all-or-none phenomenon; all stars looked alike. You either had one or you didn't. Human life and "normal" appearance are (and have always been) far more complex. Almost from the beginning of recorded time, humans have been concerned with form and, in some cultures, would abandon or kill unwanted infants, particularly those with visible birth defects, such as a cleft lip. Although abandoned infants were, on occasion, adopted to be raised as slaves, those with obvious disfigurement were not acceptable. Oedipus, that character of profound literary and psychoanalytic note, was purposely altered by his mother, the queen, who wrapped his ankles so that his feet would swell, anticipating that when abandoned he would not be adopted (*Oedipus* means "swollen feet"). Deformity and disfigurement also followed injury or disease. Leprosy, for instance, often destroyed the bridge of the nose, making a person suffering from this frightful disease apparent to all. Amputation of part or all of the nose was a common punishment for some crimes, leaving the criminal's offense visible to all. Then, and even now in much of the world, those with visible deformity were considered freaks and relegated to the margins of society.

The term *plastic* is derived from the Greek word for "shape" or "form." Almost from the beginning of surgery, there were attempts to make persons look more "normal." Efforts to repair lost noses using tissue from the cheek date back more than 2,500 years to India. In the fifteenth century it was reported that the Branca family of Sicily could restore lost noses but kept the method secret, much as the Chamberlains in Britain had done with the obstetrical forceps. (Such stories of secrecy and selfishness deprived untold numbers of women the increased safety the forceps would have provided in delivery.) Sharing of new information, although now standard in medicine, was not always readily practiced. It is therefore notable that in the sixteenth century in Bologna, Gaspare Tagliacozzi published the technique of rebuilding the nose using tissue from the arm. Although the Church deplored his technique, his descriptions and illustrations of the operation gave it to the world. Later, J. C. Carpue of Britain wrote of a method to "restore a lost nose" using tissue from the forehead. Surgeons required three millennia to achieve three painful advances in reconstruction: use of the cheek, the arm, and the forehead to rebuild a nose. Heroic patients underwent these procedures, by daring surgeons, *before* the invention of anesthesia, all in an effort to look normal. I am fortunate to be part of an era that in the last thirty to forty years produced more advances in reconstruction than had occurred in the prior history of the world.

The beginning of the twentieth century ushered in modern reconstructive surgery, which became possible because of advances in anesthesia and attention to control of infection by aseptic techniques and, later, antibiotics. Advances in plastic surgery can be specifically dated to wars and the efforts to rebuild those injured in battle. World War I, fought in trenches, had many injuries to the face and jaws (maxillofacial injuries); and World War II produced disproportionate numbers of injuries to extremities, particularly the hands, and burns. My own teacher of plastic surgery fought in World War II and was later trained by the famous Sir Harold Gillies, modern father of our specialty. The concept of "board-certified" dates to the establishment of a review board in 1939 to establish criteria for training in the specialty and to examine and certify those who are so knowledgeable and skilled. We plastic surgeons were the new restorers of lost noses and other stars.

The day I was allowed to dissect the tissue of a human being in our medical school anatomy laboratory, I was changed forever and there was no turning back. When I participated as a student in my first operation, I felt a visceral excitement and emotion all but unmatched in my lifetime. Surgery was an endless thrill and awesome privilege. During my training in general surgery, I was what my chief of plastic surgery later called a "bucket surgeon." My training had emphasized removal of tumors of the breast and internal organs, and surgery on various inflammatory diseases of intestines. At the end of most operations, there was ultimately a specimen in "the bucket." It was only after an introduction to plastic surgery that the possibility of building or rebuilding the tissues of the body presented itself to me.

Into the Sneetch world came Sylvester McMonkey McBean. McBean had a very "peculiar machine"; for three dollars each, Plain-Bellied Sneetches went in and then popped out of the machine with bellies that now had "stars upon thars."

Into my world came plastic surgery. What an amazing and beautiful career I had of learning and teaching others how to use and improve the metaphorical star machine! While still in training, I transplanted a dog's abdominal wall tissue to the dog's neck by reestablishing vascular continuity. Although Alexis Carrel had transplanted kidneys in rats and our plastic-surgery colleague Joseph Murray would later transplant a kidney between identical twins, this tissue transfer on the dog was special. It was the first application of those microsurgical techniques that are now used in breast reconstruction, reconstruction of wounds of the limbs, and, in 2008, the first successful facial transplantations. Although I performed simpler procedures and wrote about the historical evolution of orbital surgery, I never had the vision of Paul Tessier to make craniofacial surgery the ultimate star machine of my generation.

Finally, I spent most of my career addressing the special problems of burned patients, their susceptibility to infection, and their special needs in reconstruction of their burn scars. Perhaps there is no more devastating loss of a star than being burned, particularly since so many burns are in children and so many could have been prevented.

What seemed common to all these efforts was the goal of establishing or restoring a semblance or facsimile of "normal." Rarely was the reconstructed tissue the visual equivalent of normal, much less beautiful. For many patients this was satisfactory, and for those who started with nothing, a little became a lot. But we humans have always desired more. Those Sneetches who originally had the stars were dismayed when the Plain-Bellied Sneetches also suddenly had stars. To confirm their superiority, the original Star-Bellies chose to have their stars removed, until they encountered a vicious cycle of "on again, off again stars." At no time did Dr. Seuss consider the possibility that maybe the Sneetches might have wished to make their stars a little bigger, or have circles around them, or even have two or three stars. Those wishes bring me to perhaps the most visible and commonly addressed issue in modern plastic surgery: aesthetic surgery, the surgery to improve the appearance of otherwise normal tissue. To not only rebuild a breast removed for cancer but also alter the size of an otherwise normal breast. To alter the normal processes of aging to provide a younger and healthier appearance. To not only build a nose from scratch but also improve the appearance of an otherwise normal nose. Ah, how my generation of plastic surgeons improved on McBean's star machine.

Like most of my generation and those following, I was almost thirty-five years old by the time I finished medical school, graduate training in surgery/plastic surgery, and military service with the Navy/Marine Corps. Thirty-two years later, at age sixty-seven, I retired from clinical practice. To some this might seem like a relatively short career, and yet I practiced longer than many. The average retirement age for surgeons is now about fifty-nine. The issues of compensation, frustration with bureaucracy, insurance, government regulation, threats, and costs of litigation account for this attrition, which represents an unconscionable premature loss of talent and experience for society.

My retirement from clinical practice, which in the last few years involved mostly burn care, was not premature; the time had arrived. I have subsequently had the privilege of earning a degree in religious studies and am now teaching religion and ethics (particularly applied to sports) at two universities. Retirement has provided me with a perspective that only time and distance can offer.

Historically, those with deformity and disfigurement have been devalued. The surgery of appearance, such as restoring noses, much less improving the configuration of an otherwise normal nose, is still thought by many to be of less societal value than other types of surgery. In my thirty years, spent entirely in academic medicine, it was relentlessly clear that the surgery of appearance was never considered to be as important as other branches of medicine and surgery. Then and now, it was usually considered to be "unnecessary," other than perhaps by the patients in need. As the practice of medicine changes in new economic times, it seems we will encounter an environment in which resources will most likely be limited. The distribution of these resources will no doubt be determined by regulators who will, inevitably, place some perceived value on the varying needs of patients. History would predict that those who are deformed and disfigured will be devalued and their care deemed "unnecessary." The future of the surgery of all Sneetches, Star-Bellied and Plain, will be in peril.

Editor's Note: Dr. Krizek has been my teacher since I was a 23-year-old. His words are held as gospel by a generation of plastic surgeons. I'm proud to have been trained as a plastic surgeon by him.

The Third Time Around

Albert E. Cram, MD, FACS

E VERY JOURNEY has to start somewhere, and roads stretch out in all directions. My own road certainly has. My surgical career started as I observed my father, a small-town family doctor, and has taken more twists and turns than San Francisco's famous Lombard Street. I've been a general surgeon taking out gallbladders. I ended up running a burn unit. In yet another incarnation, I was chief of plastic surgery at a medical school, and (perhaps) my final role is that of a plastic surgeon in private practice.

My dad graduated from medical school in 1928, in an era without antibiotics and just a few years after the discovery of a new wonder drug they called insulin. In Burwell, Nebraska, Dad *was* the healthcare system for a small population spread over several hundred square miles of sandhills and prairie. Medical school in the 1920s was four years long. Internship paid fifteen dollars a month, lasted for eighteen months, and included training in surgical procedures such as tonsillectomy and appendectomy. It was more than a hundred miles of dirt road from Burwell to the nearest surgical specialist. There were no helicopters, no paramedics, and no CT scans. The Great Depression was tough even for doctors, and in World War II Dad became a captain in the medical corps in the North African and then the Italian theaters.

My first memories of the physician's life are of small-town Nebraska, where I was born in 1942. During my youth I saw only the tough side: my father was on call twenty-four hours a day, seven days a week. No meal was ever eaten without at least one phone call. Countless family gatherings were interrupted for a variety of often mundane but sometimes emergent situations. It was clear to me that Dad loved his work and that his patients held him in high esteem. In a career that stretched from 1930 to the late seventies, he never had a malpractice lawsuit. But to me it all seemed too high a price to pay: the years of school, the sixty-hour workweeks, the baby deliveries in the middle of the night, and the never-ending sense of responsibility for every living human in my little world. I was hoping for something a little less demanding of my time and energy.

I aimed for a career as a lawyer, but during my junior year in college, somewhere between accounting and history, my boredom hit new levels and my dad's career choice seemed invigorating for the first time since I was a child. I mapped out my medical school required courses and not only finished college on schedule but managed to get married, have two children, and work nights in the same hospital in which my mother had trained as a nurse some thirty years earlier.

I graduated from the University of Nebraska Medical Center College of Medicine in 1969, forty-one years after my father. During those four decades, I figured the information I needed to learn was ten times what my father had learned, yet we both had four years to master it. During those years it wasn't my father's family practice I was attracted to, it was surgery. I preferred curing diseases like appendicitis with strokes of the scalpel over treating chronic diseases with medications, and so I headed east— all the way to the University of Iowa—for my residency.

After my five years of general surgery residency, I joined the United States Navy and went off to the USS *Enterprise*, where I saw most of Southeast Asia from the aircraft carrier deck. There were endless days of medical boredom punctuated by the occasional appendectomy and hand injury repairs. The Navy surprised me when they discharged me after thirteen months because the Vietnam War had ended.

After the war, I returned to Iowa City and began building the state's trauma system at the university. When one of my mentors at Iowa left his position as director of the university's Burn Treatment Center, my career took another turn. I was asked to run the center temporarily until we could recruit another director. Two years and many interviews later we still didn't have a new director, and I was enjoying the management of major burn injuries so much that I decided to keep the job.

The University of Iowa was a major medical center even in the 1980s. But like so many in that era, it had no full-time plastic surgeon on staff. As the "burn guy," I also became the "wound guy," one step closer to plastic surgery than the other general surgeons. I did complex reconstructive operations after reading articles describing them, having never actually seen them. Eventually I struck a deal with my chief. He sent me off to the University of Chicago to learn plastic surgery with the agreement that I return to Iowa for at least five years. It was as far east as a Nebraskan dare venture.

So at age forty-two I became a trainee again. Old dogs can learn new tricks, and it was more fun the second time around, despite the bad hours and lousy pay. After being a top dog in Iowa, with residents, medical students, and support staff at my call, I became a lowly resident once again. My chief in Chicago, Dr. Thomas Krizek, had a unique teaching style that you can experience firsthand by reading his chapter in this book. He captured the attention of sleepy, uninterested medical students and stimulated even old, jaded residents. And as a resident only eight years away from AARP eligibility, I was fifteen years older than the other resident, Dr. Arthur Perry, the editor of this book. Going back to residency two decades after completing medical school is fairly unusual. And in plastic surgery it may just have been unprecedented. I was a seasoned general surgeon, having had full responsibility for general surgery, burn, and reconstructive patients in Iowa. But as a resident, I was subservient to surgeons much younger than I and with much less surgical experience. Still, they had completed plastic surgery training, something I had not done. And so I became a resident again and learned how to think like, act like, and operate like a plastic surgeon. I quickly adapted to Chicago, which to me was the City of Perpetual Night. I drove to the hospital at 5:30 A.M., noting the glimmer of city lights on Lake Michigan, and returned home at 10:30 P.M., noting the glimmer of city lights on Lake Michigan. It should have been exhausting, but the wide variety of interesting surgical cases was so fascinating that it all passed too quickly.

I returned to Iowa in 1987 and began creating a plastic surgery section within the university. This wasn't the easiest task in a university that had survived without plastic surgeons for the fifty years since the birth of the specialty. But I built the section to include four full-time surgeons, all performing academically and technically difficult cases as well as teaching and performing research. In 2004 I came to another fork in the road and chose the one leading in a new direction—out of the ivory tower after nearly forty years and into the private practice of plastic surgery. Intertwining cosmetic surgery with complicated reconstructive procedures, I loved my job as chief of plastic surgery at the University of Iowa. But after seventeen years as the chief, I watched as academic medicine no longer reminded me of my dad's practice. The university had changed as managed care altered my ability to act independently as a surgeon, and so in my sixties, I began a new journey, in a private practice that emphasizes aesthetic surgery. But unlike what you see on those terrible television shows, real life as a plastic surgeon still involves running to emergency rooms to sew up little kids, dealing with midlife crises of newly wrinkled housewives, and sometimes even struggling to pay bills.

I never expected to have an affinity for aesthetic surgery when I left to study plastic surgery in Chicago. I really just wanted to learn how to fix difficult wounds. But while I was there, a strange thing occurred. I learned the value that cosmetic surgery can have in a person's life, how it can be a life-changing event, and how plastic surgeons are really the restorers of self-esteem and a sense of "whole."

It was a cold day in December when a young woman and her fifteen-year-old brother came to my cosmetic surgery resident clinic. Eddie and his sister sat patiently for an hour in a no-frills waiting room in South Chicago. They were there to see me—a not quite fully trained plastic surgeon. Eddie was a shy boy with a small chin and a large nose. Like so many other kids his age, he struggled with peer acceptance—and those peers can be brutal. He was so introverted he barely communicated with the residents and nurses in the clinic. His sister told us he was intelligent but was now failing in school. The teasing by other boys was grating on his sense of well-being. And at fifteen, he was not close to being confident enough to date girls. His sister asked us to improve his appearance to boost his confidence. I'll never forget her saying, "Please help my little brother." Eddie was in our aesthetic clinic because his family could not afford a private doctor. One of the full-time attendings at the university saw him with me and helped plan his surgery. Larry and I performed a chin implant and a rhinoplasty on Eddie, making his chin larger and his nose smaller in three hours. It was a simple outpatient procedure; he was back to school in a week. Six weeks after surgery, when he showed up for a clinic appointment, Eddie was not the same person. He was happy and confident. Even the way he walked was different. His sense of self-worth had soared. And he spoke! He made many friends in his new school and his grades improved. This physical makeover had produced a miraculous beneficial psychological effect, something that would have taken shrinks a lifetime of therapy to accomplish. And with the case of Eddie, I was hooked. Cosmetic surgery wasn't frivolous after all. Through a simple surgical procedure, years of unhappiness can be avoided and personalities can be changed.

Six months before each change in my career, I would have denied the direction of the new road ahead. But life takes those twists and turns that are hard to predict. What lies ahead? Somewhere around the next corner could be exciting new opportunity.

Editor's Note: Dr. Cram and I trained together at the University of Chicago. Despite a huge age difference, we got along like brothers. Al is an unflappable surgeon, and an innovator of surgical body-lifting techniques following massive weight loss.

The Regulatory Board

Arthur W. Perry, MD, FACS

THE PHONE CALL was innocent enough. Another plastic surgeon's secretary called to ask my nurse how we sterilize our instruments in our office. An autoclave, of course, my nurse said. And you? "My surgeon just uses rubbing alcohol to clean off instruments. Our scissors is so dirty we call it the 'dreaded scissors.'"

Did I hear that right? Another board-certified plastic surgeon was performing office surgery on patients without properly sterilizing his instruments? In the AIDS and MRSA era?

Incredulous, I wrote a letter to the New Jersey State Board of Medical Examiners. Turning in another physician is never easy, but the law is very clear. If a physician learns of a situation that endangers the welfare of the public, he has the legal obligation to report it to the Board of Medical Examiners. And operating on a patient with unclean instruments exposes every patient to potentially deadly infectious disease.

The Board's reply was equally extraordinary. Not properly sterilizing instruments may have been malpractice (a civil charge), but it did not violate board regulations or existing statutes (the law). And then the kicker: "The Board does agree with you that this is a problem. Would you like to write the standards for office sterilization for the state?"

As a plastic surgeon with a research background in surgical infection, I didn't take long long to write a set of standards that every physician must follow when sterilizing instruments in the office. My rules became New Jersey policy when the standard was published in 1992. Soon after, Kansas and Georgia asked permission to use my standards, and then the federal Occupational Safety and Health Administration (OSHA) adopted them. I was inspired.

Shortly thereafter, I was asked by the board to sit on a state committee that was charged to make in-office surgery safer. Office surgery was the rage in the 1990s, and once out of the oversight of hospitals, some physicians opted to cut corners. As a result of this sloppiness, there were many in-office deaths in New Jersey and around the country. I dug into this task, not knowing that these "simple" regulations would take over a decade to enact.

The state board is the only avenue for a doctor to influence public policy, unless he runs for public office. And so I wrote the governor asking to be appointed to the board. No luck, it turned out. Who would have guessed that you had to be a member of the sitting political party in order to volunteer for part-time public service? So I waited until a Republican was in office, and in 1995 Governor Christine Todd Whitman appointed me to a three-year term on the New Jersey State Board of Medical Examiners. The board is considered the penultimate "committee assignment" for physicians. Compared to hospital and medical society committees, the board has real power and responsibility.

Complete with a new ID and even an official parking space, I drove to Trenton, shook hands with other board members, and took my seat as a newly minted board member. In addition to making the regulations that govern the medical profession, the board is charged with the responsibility of licensing and disciplining physicians. Kind of like being the judge, jury, and executioner—all in one. An awesome responsibility, the board's primary task is to protect the public.

I took my seat at the end of a very long table. The twenty-one members of the board were seated according to seniority. I was furthest from the head of the table. The first hearing that day was for a doctor who was accused of molesting his patient. In the course of a physical examination, he told her that her pain would be lessened with massage. Inappropriate at best, criminal at worst, his ensuing massage included her breasts and genitals. She left his office in tears, went to the local police station, and filed a complaint. The police told her that it would be a "he said, she said" situation because there were no witnesses. Would she go back to the doctor with a hidden camera? She did just that and recorded forty-five minutes of tilted video evidence that the board was required to watch. So through forty-five long minutes (did I mention it lasted forty-five minutes?), twenty-one board members and a slew of deputy attorneys general and staffers watched as a woman allowed herself to be molested a second time. Needless to say, the board revoked the license of this doctor, who also then faced a criminal charge.

Much to my relief, this sort of video was never to be repeated during my tenure on the board. We did, however, see the gamut of bad medicine. From on-the-job drug abuse to dirty offices, to nonsurgeons killing patients by performing surgery, to physicians rubbing genitals against secretaries' buttocks, we saw it all. Reprimanding doctors, mandating retraining, and suspending and revoking licenses was the part of the job that wasn't much fun but was necessary to keep the public safe.

Being a member of a state board is considered prestigious. Selection is based on educational background, ideas, and a clean record with the board. But becoming a member of the board is like becoming an IRS agent: the tax cheats probably won't want to go to dinner with you. So, much to my surprise, some doctors who referred patients to me *stopped* referring after I became a member of the board. Being on the board was not a practice-building plan, I decided.

As the weeks and years went on I became an integral part of the board, and for most years I was the only surgeon. During disciplinary hearings, my standards fell back to my Harvard training. Sometimes I argued with other board members, who felt my standards were unrealistically high; they stated that doctors should be held to a "community standard."

Unlike in the 1950s, in this era of readily available education there is no reason why medical care shouldn't be up to the standards taught at the nation's best medical schools. The "community standard" is an outdated concept. Doctors shouldn't sink to the lowest standard of an existing medical community. We're not talking about carpentry here—we're talking about patients' lives. I judged other doctors based on how I would want *my* family treated. My privileged position allowed me to learn about medical problems that were never published in textbooks *or* the newspapers. I saw liposuction deaths that were avoidable and was able to integrate information I learned from these problems into everyday practice. A clinical study I performed as a result of my board experience resulted in my publishing a safer liposuction technique.

Eventually, I became chairman of a preliminary evaluation committee that processed initial complaints against doctors and ran preliminary hearings. We were the first to ask doctors "What happened?" after a complaint was filed, then recommended action to the full board. While on the board, I heavily influenced the in-office surgical standards, was the board's liaison to the electrology and cosmetology boards, and even proposed regulations for tattooing and piercing. And when the planes hit the World Trade Center on September 11 and New Jersey became a focus of the anthrax attacks, I was appointed as the bioterrorism liaison from the board to the New Jersey Department of Health, working with the state and federal government to ensure that the country was safe from a smallpox attack. A phone call from Karl Rove (then senior advisor to President George W. Bush) one night made me realize that this was not just another committee assignment.

Like the endless *Gilligan's Island* three-hour tour, my supposed three-year appointment extended more than ten years, courtesy of a reappointment by Governor Whitman and inattention from Governor James McGreevey, who may have been a little distracted before he resigned in disgrace. I gradually moved from the back of the table to the front, and for a time was an officer of the board. But after more than 368 full-day meetings (but who's counting?) that sometimes extended into the night, and a decade of dragging around stacks of paper so high that they were comical, my tenure ended, without notice but with a great sense of accomplishment.

REFLECTIONS OF A
CARDIOVASCULAR SURGEON

Denton A. Cooley, MD, FACS

A T THE BEGINNING of my career as a surgeon, I knew of
the admonitions that the heart should not be manipu-
lated I was fortunate, therefore, in being present at one of
the major milestones in a new specialty of heart surgery.

At Johns Hopkins Hospital in November 1944, I was
an assistant to Dr. Alfred Blalock in doing the first operation for treatment of tetralogy of Fallot (a congenital heart
defect that deprives the blood of oxygen), the so-called
blue-baby operation. At the dawn of modern heart surgery, this was a major stimulus to others to begin explor-
ing the possibility of cardiac manipulation and surgery.
In most of those operations in the early years, techniques

were confined to the cardiac surface, or to the major arteries off the heart. The challenge was to develop a means of operating inside the heart (intracardiac surgery) but yet to permit the repair to be done under direct vision.

We developed a rather simple pump and oxygenator in which blood was bubbled with oxygen to restore cardiac function. With this device, we became explorers in a new field of cardiac surgery. The open-heart era in surgery that followed was exciting. Almost all the operations done were considered unique and reportable, and newspaper headlines followed. Surgery for aortic aneurysms presented a challenge to surgeons. After removal of the aneurysm, reconnecting the largest artery in the body was necessary. Many ingenious techniques were developed to satisfy this purpose using fabric and biologic grafts.

In 1951 I returned to my hometown of Houston, Texas, where I joined the Baylor College of Medicine faculty. Eleven years later I chartered and founded the Texas Heart Institute for the study and treatment of diseases of the heart and blood vessels. Perhaps the most exciting event in cardiac surgery occurred in December 1967, when the first heart transplantation was performed in Cape Town, South Africa. I became involved in cardiac transplantation several months later and performed the first successful heart transplantation in the United States. This operation, which had such a spectacular result, inspired us to proceed with cardiac transplantation in the following months, with six out of the first seven patients having successful results. I led a team that developed expertise in this operation and it soon became apparent that we needed a mechanical substitute or artificial heart as a bridge to transplantation.

In April 1969, after we had performed many experimental procedures in calves to test an artificial heart, we finally had the opportunity to implant the device in a human patient. This introduced a new concept: a mechanical heart used as a temporary bridge to transplantation until a suitable donor could be obtained. The concepts and surgical procedures have been a resounding success! At the Texas Heart Institute more than one thousand heart transplants have been performed, each one representing a saved life.

The major impact on the volume of cardiac surgery began in the ensuing years when coronary bypass surgery was introduced. We became very much involved and have accumulated thousands of successful cases. My colleagues and I have performed more than 120,000 open heart procedures.

Recently, when I attended a meeting concerned with medical ethics, the moderator had some difficulty in introducing me to the audience. He said that several surgeons had been named the "father of heart surgery," but it occurred to him that perhaps I should be introduced as "a midwife to the specialty" for my role in the birth and early development of most new cardiac procedures.

The future promises to be productive, but perhaps not as exciting as the challenges of the past five decades in this field.

Editor's Note: Babe Ruth, Neil Armstrong, Albert Einstein, Denton Cooley. They're all legends—but only one is a surgeon. This story is an understated account of the beginning of cardiac surgery in the world. Dr. Cooley is responsible for revolutionizing the surgical treatment of the heart. Millions of people owe their lives to him.

About the Editor

ARTHUR W. PERRY, MD, FACS is a plastic surgeon in private practice in central New Jersey and Manhattan, New York.

While a "real surgeon," seeing patients and performing cosmetic surgery 60 hours a week, Dr. Perry has had a varied career. He received his undergraduate degree *magna cum laude* with high distinction in zoology in just three years. His medical degree was awarded with distinction in research from the Albany Medical College of Union University. He then spent three years as an intern and general surgical resident at Harvard Medical School's Beth Israel Hospital in Boston, and a year as the burn fellow at The New York Hospital/Cornell Medical Center. His plastic and reconstructive surgery residency was then completed at the University of Chicago, where he was Chief Resident in 1986–87. Prior to joining the full-time faculty of the University of Medicine and Dentistry of New Jersey–Robert Wood Johnson Medical School, he performed a cosmetic surgery fellowship with Drs. Baker and Gordon in Miami.

Dr. Perry has been named to the "Best Doctors in the New York area" book each year since 1999 and has been named to *New York Magazine's* Top Doctors list in 2007 and 2008.

Dr. Perry left the full-time faculty but still teaches residents and medical students at Robert Wood Johnson, where he is a Clinical Associate Professor of Plastic Surgery. For fourtenn years he was also a Clinical Associate at the University of Pennsylvania School of Medicine and he now collaborates with the Cornell/Columbia plastic surgery residency program. For his teaching, he was awarded the Volunteer Faculty Award for outstanding service at Robert Wood Johnson. He has also won two national awards for his plastic surgery research and has published many scientific papers and medical chapters.

Dr. Perry spent a decade on New Jersey's State Board of Medical Examiners and received the Distinguished Service Award for Outstanding Contributions to Plastic Surgery and to the New Jersey State Board of Medical Examiners from the New Jersey Society of Plastic Surgeons.

A writer since college and medical school (where he was the founding editor of the school newspaper), Dr. Perry's first book, *Are You Considering Cosmetic Surgery?*, was published in 1997. His second book, *Straight Talk about Cosmetic Surgery* won *Foreword Magazine's* Award for the top health book of 2007. His third book, *You – Being Beautiful*, co-authored with Drs. Michael Roizen and Mehmet Oz and Ted Spiker, Craig Wynett, and Lisa Oz, was on the *New York Times* bestseller list for 10 weeks.

Dr. Perry has been the host of a plastic surgery show on radio station WOR in New York for four years. He has co-hosted the nationally syndicated "You the Owners Manual" radio show with Dr. Roizen for two years. His one-minute plastic surgery vignettes "Looking in the Mirror with Dr. Arthur Perry" are broadcast throughout the U.S. on the WOR radio network.

About the Contributors

MARK B. ANDERSON, MD, FACS, is Chief of Cardiac Surgery, Director of the Minimally Invasive Cardiac Surgery Program and Associate Professor of Surgery at UMDNJ-Robert Wood Johnson Medical School. He received his medical degree at New York Medical College in Valhalla, New York. He obtained his residency training in general surgery at Lenox Hill Hospital in New York and Cardiothoracic surgery at the University of California, San Diego. Dr. Anderson has successfully restarted Robert Wood Johnson University Hospital's heart transplant program and broadened its scope to support and treat heart failure patients with the latest medical and surgical therapies, including ventricular assist devices. Dr. Anderson has published many scholarly articles and presents at many scientific conferences. He is constantly searching for new ways to make minimally invasive surgery a viable option for cardiac patients. In April 2005, Dr. Anderson received the Harvey E. Nussbaum, MD Distinguished Service Award from the American Heart Association.

NEAL S. CAYNE, MD, FACS, is the Director of New York University's Endovascular Surgery program. He received an Engineering degree from the University of Michigan in 1991, then matriculated at New York Medical College, where he was inducted into the Alpha Omega Alpha Medical Honor Society. In 1995, he began his five-year General Surgery Training at Montefiore Medical Center/Albert Einstein College of Medicine, where he remained for his two-year Vascular and Endovascular fellowship. Dr. Cayne is now an assistant professor of surgery at NYU, specializing in vascular surgery. He has published in many areas, including abdominal aortic aneurysms and minimally invasive vascular procedures. He is currently the principal investigator for multiple clinical trials involving new devices for carotid stenting and the treatment of abdominal and thoracic aortic aneurysms.

CHRISTOPHER COPPOLA, MD, MC, USAF, is a pediatric surgeon in Texas. His training includes medical school at Johns Hopkins, residency at Yale, and fellowship at the Children's National Medical Center. He has served in the United States Air Force Medical Corps, and is a veteran of Operation Iraqi Freedom. He has completed humanitarian missions to Brazil and Haiti. He and his family enjoy the high-tech sport of geocaching, as well as roaming parks and trails in their lightly modified Wrangler.

DENTON A. COOLEY, MD, FACS, is president-emeritus and surgeon-in-chief of the Texas Heart Institute at St.

Luke's Episcopal Hospital in Houston, Texas. Dr. Cooley graduated from Johns Hopkins School of Medicine in Baltimore in 1944 (AOA) and completed his surgical residency under Dr. Alfred Blalock. Upon completing his residency, he joined Mr. Russell Brock at the Brompton Hospital in London, England, where he was a senior surgical registrar. After completing his training, he became a full-time faculty member of Baylor College of Medicine in Houston; he resigned in 1969 to become surgeon-in-chief of the Texas Heart Institute. Dr. Cooley is a member of more than 50 professional societies and was president of the Society of Thoracic Surgeons. Among his more than 120 honors and awards are the National Medal of Technology; the National Medal of Freedom, the nation's highest civilian award; the Theodore Roosevelt award, given by the National Collegiate Athletic Association to a varsity athlete who has achieved national recognition in his profession; and the Rene Leriche Prize, the highest honor of the International Surgical Society. Throughout his 65-year career, Dr. Cooley has been a leading contributor to the evolution, technological development, and practice of cardiac surgery. He is known for developing techniques to treat congenital heart disease in infants and children, popularizing the use of non-blood prime for cardiopulmonary bypass, implanting the first total artificial heart implant in a human, and performing the first successful heart transplant in the United States. He and his team have performed over 100,000 open heart operations, and he has published more than 1,200 peer-reviewed scientific publications.

ALBERT E. CRAM, MD, FACS, graduated from the University of Nebraska College of Medicine in 1969, and completed general surgery training at the University of Iowa College of Medicine in 1974. After completing a military tour of duty as a surgeon aboard the USS Enterprise, he returned there as a trauma surgeon, and later served as head of the University of Iowa Burn Center. During the late 70s and early 80s he served as chairman of the Govenor's Emergency Medical Services Advisory Committee and helped develop the early paramedic, helicopter, and emergency medical care system in the state of Iowa. In 1985 he became a resident again, this time in the plastic surgery training program at the University of Chicago. Now retired from academic practice, Dr. Cram is currently in private practice in plastic surgery.

IAN G. DORWARD, MD, graduated from Washington University in St. Louis School of Medicine, and is currently completing his residency in neurological surgery. His medical stories have appeared in *Bellevue Literary Review*, *Ars Medica*, and a special edition of *The Lancet*. He and his wife, a dermatologist, are expecting their first child.

GEORGE A. FIELDING, MDMD, FRCS, FRACS, associate professor of surgery at New York University's school of medicine, is a pioneer in laparoscopic and bariatric surgery. Dr. Fielding studied medicine at the University of Queensland, graduating in 1979, and completed his medical training at the Royal Brisbane Hospital. He trained in Australia, Britain, and Switzerland, and has actively pursued teaching laparoscopic surgery to physicians in the United States, Japan, and various other Asian and European countries. To date, he has performed more than 4,500 bariatric surgeries, and has extensive experience operating on "super" obese patients. Dr. Fielding is a fellow of the Royal Australian College of Surgeons and Britain's Royal College of Surgeons. In addition, he is a member of the American Society of Bariatric Surgeons, the Society of Surgery for the Alimentary Tract, the Society of American Gastrointestinal Endoscopic Surgeons, and the International Hepato-Pancreato-Biliary Association. He has published more than 150 journal articles, abstracts, and book chapters, and has appeared in numerous venues for the lay public, including *The Today Show, The Jane Pauley Show, The New York Times, The Montel Williams Show* and the *New York Post.*

YUMAN FONG, MD, FACS, is a Liver and Pancreatic Surgeon specializing in the treatment of cancers of those organs. After graduating from Brown University with a degree in medieval literature, he attended medical school at the Cornell University Medical College. He did his residency and fellowship training at the New York Hospital-Cornell Medical Center, and at the Memorial Sloan-Kettering Cancer Center. He currently holds the Murray F. Brennan Chair in surgery, and is the co-director of the Center for Image Guided Interventions at the Memorial Sloan-Kettering Cancer Center. In his spare time he coaches youth athletics, and recently coached both his daughter Sandy at the Beijing Olympics and his daughter Danielle at the Beijing Paralympics.

BRUCE L. GEWERTZ, MD, FACS, is Surgeon-in-Chief, Chair of the Department of Surgery and Vice-President for Interventional Services at Cedars-Sinai Health System in Los Angeles. Previously, he was on the faculty at the University of Chicago for 25 years, serving as the Dallas B. Phemister Professor and chair of the department of surgery from 1992 until 2006. He was educated at Pennsylvania State University and Jefferson Medical College in the combined BS-MD five year program. He trained in general and vascular surgery at the University of Michigan. Dr. Gewertz is the author of more than 200 original articles, book chapters and books. Dr. Gewertz has received numerous awards for his basic investigations and teaching and was selected Outstanding Science Alumnus by Pennsylvania State University in 2003. Dr. Gewertz enjoys fitness training, skiing and golf. He and his wife Diane most value time at home and on the road with their five children, grandchildren, and energetic Wheaten Terrier.

JAMES S. COYDOS, MD, FACS, is an associate professor of surgery at the University of Medicine and Dentistry of New Jersey-Robert Wood Johnson Medical School, and director of the melanoma and soft tissue sarcoma program at the Cancer Institute of New Jersey—the state's only comprehensive cancer center designated by the National

Cancer Institute. He received his medical degree from UMDNJ-Robert Wood Johnson Medical School. Dr. Goydos completed his residency training at The University of Connecticut, followed by a fellowship at the University of Pittsburgh in surgical oncology and biological therapy. Dr. Goydos' main clinical interests are treating melanoma and soft tissue sarcomas with the latest treatment options, including state-of-the-art clinical trials and surgical procedures

ROBERT T. GRANT, MD, MSC, FACS, is the Plastic Surgeon-in-Chief for the combined divisions of Plastic Surgery at New York-Presbyterian Hospital, the University Hospitals of Columbia, and Cornell University. He is also an associate clinical professor of surgery at Columbia University, College of Physicians and Surgeons and an adjunct associate professor of plastic surgery at Cornell's Weill Medical College. A New York native, Dr. Grant received his medical degree from Albany Medical College, and completed his general surgery and plastic surgery residencies at the New York Hospital-Cornell Medical Center. Board-certified in General Surgery and Plastic Surgery, Dr. Grant is a member of the American Association of Plastic Surgeons, the American Society for Aesthetic Plastic Surgery, and the American Society of Plastic Surgeons. He is a fellow of the American College of Surgeons. In addition to numerous local and national radio and TV appearances, Dr. Grant has been included in *New York* magazine's list of "Best Doctors in New York."

MEGHANN KAISER, MD, FACS, is finishing her residency training in general surgery at the University of California, Irvine. She has written several poems, short stories and essays which appear in *Body Language: Poems of the Medical Training Experience, The Legible Script National Literal Journal, Plexus Journal of Arts and Humanities, The American College of Emergency Physicians Medical Humanities Section Newsletter, Family, System & Health Journal,* and the *Journal of General Internal Medicine,* among others. She and her husband live in Orange County with their Yorkshire Terrier and two parrots.

RICHARD C. KARL, MD, FACS, is is a native of New York, where he received his medical degree from Cornell University in 1970. He completed his general surgery residency and post doctoral research training at the Washington University School of Medicine, Barnes Hospital in St. Louis. He served on the faculty at the University of Chicago as assistant and associate professor of surgery. In 1984, Dr. Karl was appointed the founding medical director of the H. Lee Moffitt Cancer Center and Research Institute, where he implemented the Interdisciplinary Gastrointestinal Tumor Program, served as Chief of Surgery, and created the surgical oncology fellowship program. Along with his academic pursuits, Dr. Karl is an active pilot and a contributing editor and columnist for Flying magazine. He has combined his two lifelong loves, surgery and flying, by founding the Surgical Safety Institute. His first book, *Across the Redline, Stories from the Surgical Life,* was published in 2002.

THOMAS J. KRIZEK, MD, FACS, is a graduate of the Marquette University School of Medicine. He trained in general and plastic surgery at University Hospital of Cleveland. He served on the full-time faculty at Johns Hopkins, and then as Chief of Plastic Surgery at Yale, Columbia-Presbyterian, the University of Southern California, the University of Chicago and the University of South Florida. He has also served as Chair of Surgery and Interim Dean at the University of Chicago. He is the former First Vice-President of the American College of Surgeons and past president of American Association of Plastic Surgeons, American Association for Hand Surgery, and Plastic Surgery Research Council. He is the author or co-author of several books, dozens of chapters, and more than 200 peer-reviewed papers. Since retiring from surgery, has earned a Master's degree in Religious Studies (Ethics), and is an adjunct professor of Religious Studies at University of South Florida and Saint Leo University.

SUSAN M. LOVE, MD, FACS, MBA, has dedicated her professional life to the eradication of breast cancer. As president of the Dr. Susan Love Research Foundation, she oversees an active research program centered on breast cancer prevention. She is a clinical professor of surgery at UCLA's David Geffen School of Medicine; founder of Windy Hill Medical, a breast cancer drug device company; and founder and senior partner in LLuminari, a multimedia women's health company. She is best known as a trusted guide to women worldwide through her books and website. *Dr. Susan Love's Breast Book* has been termed "the bible for women with breast cancer" by *The New York Times*. Dr. Love received her medical degree from SUNY Downstate Medical Center in New York, and completed her surgical training at Boston's Beth Israel Hospital. She founded the Faulkner Breast Center in Boston and the Revlon UCLA Breast Center in Los Angeles. She has a business degree from the Executive MBA program at UCLA's Anderson School. In 1996 she retired from the active practice of surgery, to dedicate her time to the urgent pursuit of finding the cause and prevention of breast cancer.

JANE E. MILLER, MD, FACOG, received her baccalaurate degree in Gallic Letters with honors from Yale University. She received her medical degree from the State University of New York Downstate Medical Center in 1978. Dr. Miller completed a postdoctoral fellowship in Psychiatry at Yale University School of Medicine before attending the residency programs in Obstetrics and Gynecology at Harvard University and the University of Tennessee. She returned to Downstate Medical Center to complete her fellowship in Reproductive Endocrinology and Infertility in 1989. She served as director of the Reproductive Endocrinology division at Newark Beth Israel Medical Center before opening the North Hudson I.V.F. Center for Fertility and Gynecology in 1995. She is board certified in both Reproductive Endocrinology and Obstetrics and Gynecology.

A. JOHN POPP, MD, FACS, is a passionate educator who enjoys training the next generation of neurological surgeons. He recently moved to Boston, Massachusetts to join the faculty of Brigham and Women's Hospital and Harvard University. Previously, he had spent his entire medical career at Albany Medical Center where he completed his neurosurgical residency, and ultimately became the chairman of the department of surgery. In 2004 the Schaffer Foundation honored Dr. Popp by endowing the A. John Popp Chair in Neurosurgery at Albany Medical Center. Dr. Popp has been a member of the American Board of Neurological Surgery, and has served as President of the American Association of Neurological Surgery and the Society of Neurological Surgeons. Currently, Dr. Popp is the president of the World Academy of Neurological Surgeons and serves on the Residency Review Committee for Neurological Surgery.

WILLIAM S. SILEN, MD, FACS, is a graduate of the University of California (San Francisco) School of Medicine, where he also received his surgical training. Dr. Silen served in the Department of Surgery at UCSF from 1960–1966, at which time he was recruited to become the Johnson & Johnson Professor of Surgery at Harvard Medical School, and Chairman of Surgery at the Beth Israel Hospital. He occupied the latter position until 1995, when he became Associate Dean for Faculty Development and Diversity at the Harvard Medical School, a position from which he retired in 2002. He continues to teach Harvard Medical Students to this day as Emeritus Professor of Surgery, and has won many teaching awards throughout his career. Dr. Silen has headed the Society for Surgery of the Alimentary Tract, the Boston Surgical Society, and the American Gastroenterological

Society. He was awarded the Julius Friedenwald Medal by the latter society and was made an Honorary Fellow of the Royal College of Surgeons of England in 1992.

RONALD S. WEISS, MD is a board certified ophthalmologist in private practice in the Chicago metro area. He also is an Assistant Professor of Ophthalmology at Rush University Medical Center. He received his undergraduate degree at Emory University in Atlanta and his medical degree at Northwestern University in Chicago. He completed his ophthalmology residency at The University of Chicago where he participated in ophthalmic research and presented at national meetings. An avid contemporary art collector, he lives with his wife and son in Chicago.

LARRY ZACHARY, MD, FACS, is a plastic and reconstructive surgeon at the University of Chicago, where he is an associate professor of surgery. As the director of plastic surgery at Weiss Memorial Hospital in Chicago, he specializes in body contouring after massive weight loss, and digital sympathectomy in the hand for patients with collagen vascular diseases such as scleroderma or SLE. He received his bachelor's degree from the University of Illinois Champaign, and his medical degree from the Chicago Medical School. He trained in general surgery at the University of Chicago and then plastic surgery at Wayne State University, followed by a hand fellowship at the Raymond Curtis Hand Center in Baltimore. He married his high school sweetheart and has three wonderful children. His parents where Holocaust survivors.

SHARE YOUR STORIES WITH KAPLAN PUBLISHING

KAPLAN PUBLISHING, A leading educational resource for doctors, would like to feature your story in an upcoming anthology in the Kaplan Voices: Doctors series. Please share the stories behind the relationships, the experiences, and the issues you've encountered in your medical career—whether you work in a bustling hospital, a rural clinic, private practice, or anywhere in between.

Entertaining and educational, inspirational and practical, each Kaplan Voices: Doctors anthology features true, first-person stories written by doctors themselves, revealing the person behind the white coat.

For writers' guidelines or more information, please contact Kaplan Publishing by email at *kaplanvoicesdoctors@ gmail.com*, or write to us at:

Kaplan Voices: Doctors editor
Kaplan Publishing
1 Liberty Plaza, 24th Floor
New York, NY 10006

Preview

THE REAL LIFE OF A PEDIATRICIAN

Perri Klass, MD

Editor

THE CARE OF STRANGERS

Rachel Kowalsky, MD

A BROTHER AND SISTER have run away from home—or
at least, they wandered away from their grandmother
in the Bronx and took the subway 17 stops, exiting at South
Street Seaport. They were found climbing over a railing to
get a better look at the boats. The brother, Rafael, hands
thrust deep into his pockets, is seven. His sister, Laura,
is four. She wears a raggedy sundress and pink sequined
shoes. Oblivious to the quorum of cops and case workers
their presence has summoned, they were ogling the fish
in the seaport's fish tank.

Their grandmother arrives in the emergency department. She is thin, anxious. She wears thick glasses and
thick heels. I break the news to her—we've had to call
ACS, the Administration for Children's Services, to inves-
tigate the family. Even if the children didn't run away—

even if they only wandered off—they were improperly supervised.

The woman is indignant, frowning at me over her glasses. "We are *buena gente*—good people. You don't know anything about us!"

She's right; I don't know them. In my job as a pediatric emergency physician, I care for thousands of children and families in a year, entering their lives at critical moments and exiting just as quickly. While many patients develop a relationship with their doctor over months and years, a typical ER shift is between 8 and 12 hours—about as long as it takes to fly cross-country, charge a battery, or marinate a chicken. It takes longer for paint to dry on the hospital walls.

The grandmother is interviewed by the ACS social worker. The office door is closed, but I can still hear the escalating emotion from down the hall. Through the shouting and crying, I catch that phrase again: *buena gente.* When she emerges, the grandmother is crying. Laura, the four-year-old, pulls herself away from the fish tank, rushes over, drapes her arms around the old woman's neck, and then starts to cry herself. The woman and child add their tears to the general din of the ER. The medical student I am working with looks at me, distraught. "Maybe we shouldn't have called ACS."

I have a set of rules for taking care of strangers, and I lecture the student about Rule Number One: *Treat every family the same.* In this frenetic setting, I will never learn whether a family is *buena gente* or not, so I have to do the same thing for every little wanderer: call ACS. If the children had strayed from a picnic on the well-heeled Upper East Side, I'd have to do the same (and I have).

Then, because I have a few moments (and the medical student is a captive audience), I share Rule Number Two: *Learn one thing from each patient.* Rafael, the seven-year-old, has a benign heart murmur. I tell her to go and listen to it. That way, when she hears an abnormal murmur, she will know the difference. "See?" I expound. "You'll never see Rafael again, but he will influence your practice for years to come."

Rules one and two are basic. Anyone who went to medical school in the last century has been lectured on both of these topics. The more difficult task, when caring for strangers, is to inject humanity into these brief encounters—to pop in and out of people's lives with grace. Thirty minutes later, when my shift ends, I make an attempt. The children and their grandmother are sitting miserably in an alcove, situated directly between me and the door. "Good-bye," I say, standing uncertainly before them. Nobody looks up. I kneel down to Laura's eye level and offer her a sticker. She scowls at me. I accept my defeat.

The other rule of caring for strangers is one I learned as a resident in pediatrics. It was routine to cross-cover patients, or to care for a patient briefly, usually overnight or on a weekend. On weekdays, each patient had a primary resident, a resident who knew the patient well and was responsible for his or her care. But, despite being called "resident," no doctor truly lives in the hospital—

and when the primary doctor went home, somebody had to assume care of those patients. This is true in essentially every hospital in the country, and it's why the cross-cover role exists. Cross-cover doctors, like ER doctors, must take care of children they do not know.

When I was a resident, we had systems in place to make cross-coverage as seamless as possible. For example, each patient had a weekly log with a column for each day of the week. Each day we recorded the vital signs and lab results, the child's medications and diet specifications, and any important events that had occurred. When we "signed out" a patient to the cross-cover, we handed that doctor the log. It became all-important—the patient's whole illness distilled into a few lines of text.

Despite all the organization, cross-coverage was always a delicate situation. Entering a child's hospital course *in medias res* felt like opening a novel to a random page, or entering a movie theater halfway through the film. I learned to ask a lot of questions at sign-out so that I would never walk into a patient's room unprepared. And I became used to hearing "you don't know my son," or "you don't know what works for my daughter." Experienced parents would even say, as I came by to introduce myself, "I know—you're just cross-covering."

And then, a resident's nightmare: I was cross-covering Amanda Lopez the night she died. Amanda (not her real name) had a rare and virulent form of childhood leukemia. She was DNR (Do Not Resuscitate) and ALOC (Altered Level of Care). The latter meant that we were not to do anything invasive or painful, such as draw blood or put in IVs. She was to receive comfort measures only.

Boyd, my co-resident, signed her out to me. Amanda's primary, Sam, was post-call—he had worked overnight the night before, going home at 11:00 A.M. So Boyd had covered Amanda. And now she was mine: double cross-coverage. She had been febrile all day, lapsing in and out of consciousness, her blood pressure falling. Boyd told me she was going to die. In fact, he had actually started the necessary paperwork for me: the death certificate, the organ donation papers, and the Event Note on the computer—the "event" being death. This is how it read: "Amanda is a 6-year-old female with leukemia. Status: post multiple rounds of chemotherapy, now with end-stage disease and presumed sepsis, on ALOC." I could write the rest later.

Amanda liked to wear ponchos. Her favorite was a nubby cream-colored poncho with navy stripes; it was way too big for her tiny body. I knew her, but not well, the way I knew the kids in my apartment building. She had been in the hospital a long time. Her log had weeks and weeks worth of papers stapled together, but since she'd become ALOC, not much was written there. She had hollow cheeks, large, lovely eyes, and a wise, pointed chin. She was very close with her oncologist and with Sam, her primary—but neither of them was there. I was there.

I introduced myself to Amanda's parents. I said I was their doctor for the night. I asked whether Amanda was comfortable and if they needed anything. Amanda's mom asked whether Sam, her primary resident, was around. I said no. He was actually at a wedding, but I couldn't bring myself to say this. She nodded. I suppose on the scale of disappointments, this final one was small. She asked me for a glass of water for Amanda. *Ice?* I asked. *No thanks.* I stood around for a bit, watching her offer the water to Amanda. I remember that the girl's lips were dry, that she didn't drink anything, and that her mom carefully applied some lip balm. Amanda lay on her side, propped up on pillows, a nasal cannula delivering oxygen with a soft whir. Her parents lay in bed too—one on either side of her. Nobody spoke to me or looked at me, so I left the room.

If Amanda's life was a novel, I was a minor character—a character without lines. I sat at the nurse's station, wondering what I could do for her. My pager went off all night, calling me to other rooms and other patients, but I kept returning to the desk outside Amanda's room. "Do you think they need me?"

Amanda's nurse shook her head. "Best to leave them alone."

It was torture not to go in the room. Shouldn't I know the patient whose final Event Note I was to write? Shouldn't there be a moment of connection? Well, I had brought her a cup of water. Somehow that made me feel better.

I checked on Amanda twice more. The first time, she was cuddling with her mother. The second time, she appeared to be asleep. An hour or two later, her nurse called me. "I think she passed," she said. She was crying. Another nurse hugged her. I stood awkwardly, my hands in the pockets of my white coat. "Go on in," she said. "You have to pronounce her."

So that was my job—to listen to Amanda's quiet chest and confirm that she was gone. I put my stethoscope over her heart and listened for a long time. When I looked up, both parents were watching me. It was a strange moment, the three of us in the room with Amanda. I opened my mouth to speak, but they cut me off. They reached for each other. And that was the end of the story.

From Amanda, I learned Rule Number Three: *family first*. I don't think her parents remember me. They probably remember Sam, and their favorite nurse. I was just the one with the stethoscope, at the end—an extra in Amanda's story, and the story of her family.

But in my own story, Amanda is a prominent figure. Because of her, I learned Rule Number Four: *12 hours is just the beginning*. Because I still think about Amanda Lopez, and it's five years later.

Don't give up. The last rule, Rule Number Five. It's weeks later, and I am back in the ER with another medical student, telling him what I like about my job. The level of acuity, the interesting cases, the varied age groups. The many dramas, big and small, that come through my door each day. The medical student plans to go into General Pediatrics because, he says, he likes the continuity of care. He wants to get to know his patients.

I defend my profession. Children with respiratory illness often come back for a "resp check"—a second visit—and babies with fevers commonly are brought back to the ER for a follow-up visit as well. If we put in stitches, we usually take them out. I enjoy these reunions, the familiar faces, the "how are you doing?"

And even though there are many patients we never see again, I tell the student, *don't give up.* After all, a lot can be accomplished in just a few hours. Parties start and end. Entire weather systems change. Shakespeare's plays are just hours long, and think of all that happens there—people fall in love, wage war, return from exile. Kingdoms fall.

And, can you believe it? That same day, I bump into the grandmother at the end of my shift. We are both in the lobby, trying to exit the hospital through the revolving door. There are several people ahead of us, and we wait awkwardly together.

Finally, she nods at me.

"The kids?" I ask, looking around. She tells me she is here alone, visiting a sick relative.

"How are they?"

"*Malcriados.*" Poorly behaved.

"I'm sorry..." I begin.

She enters the revolving door, waving away my apology. "The woman came from ACS, she checked the house, she talked to us—and she left. She saw we were good people."

"I try to treat every family the same," I say, defending myself as I stumble through the door behind her.

She stands and faces me in the bright sunlight. Then, she surprises me. "You did the right thing," she says. "If somebody had done that for my brother and me when we were young, it might have saved his life." And just like that, she strides off in her thick heels. The whole conversation is two minutes from start to finish—about as long as it takes to adjust to the winter light, shake my head, and watch her disappear down the broad avenue.